Discovering
Life After Alzheimer's

A 26,000 Mile Motorcycle
Ride Across America
Del Lonnquist

Cover design by Del Lonnquist

Published by MtSky Press
P.O. Box 6444 Helena, Mt. 59604

For information contact:
DelLonnquist@Gmail.com

All rights reserved.
ISBN:0978696360
ISBN-13: 978-0978696368

DEDICATION

To Lois

It was a long ride,
and we rode it together

ACKNOWLEDGMENTS

The Lonnquist Family
Children
Grand Children
Great Grand Children

They were always there

CONTENTS

Epilogue
Helpful ideas For Caregivers

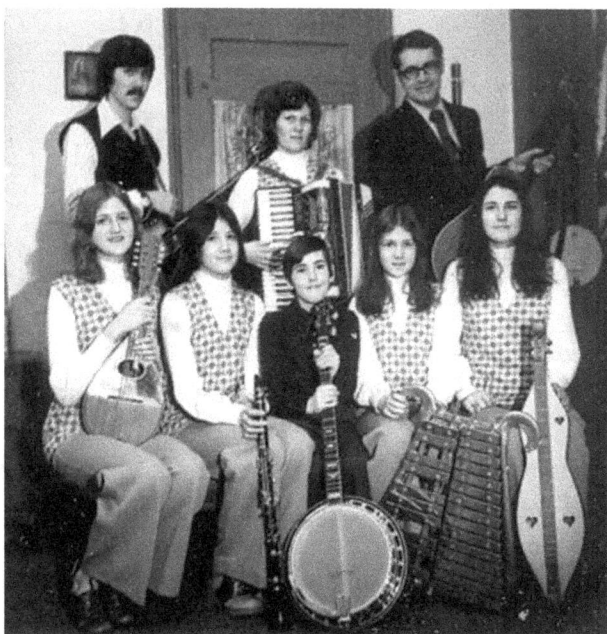

BACK: ALLEN LOIS DEL
FRONT: DIANA JANIS ROGER JONI LINDA

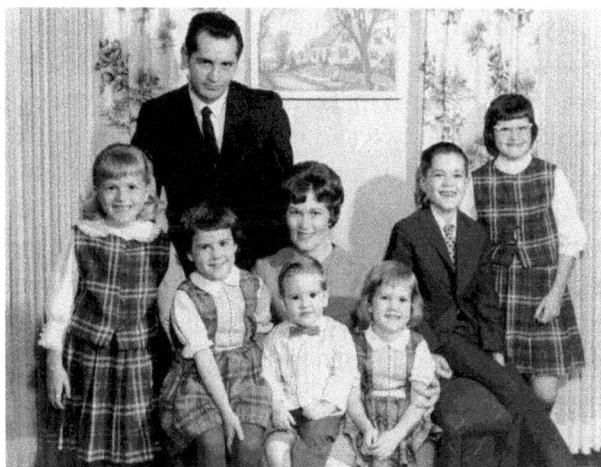

DEL DIANA JANIS LOIS ROGER
JONI ALLEN LINDA

1 - THE ACCIDENT

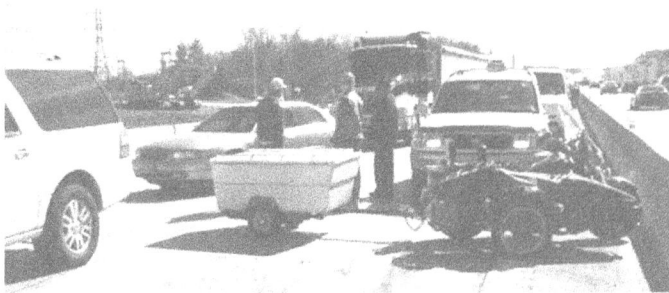

Skidded Sideways To A Stop

There were four lanes of traffic merging into three lanes and traveling at 70 MPH when the young guy in lane one hit the construction project barricade.

Three barrels of sand seemed to explode and the sand sprayed high in the air.

He slammed on his brakes and skidded sideways clear across all four lanes. I was in lane three and hit the brakes hard as he skidded in front of me.

My motorcycle and sidecar did a slide out skidding sideways as the Mini Mate trailer jackknifed behind me. As I was about to make contact with the young guys car the vehicle in lane two slid over to lane three and T-Boned the kids car pushing it away from me and it ended up some 15 or 20 feet ahead of me in the middle of the road. A young guy driving a pick up truck was in lane four and when I skidded into his lane he braked hard and somehow was able to stop four or five feet back without hitting me. He jumped out of his truck and ran to me calling out, "Are you okay, Are you okay"

I assured him I was fine and he said, "Mister, the sign says you're 80 years old, but I don't care how old you are, that was one helluva a piece of riding you just did. When you began to jackknife I thought you were a goner."

"I told you this would happen, I told you!"
That's what Lois would have said if she had been there.
And that's what she did say that time years ago when I hit
the deer while riding my motorcycle to work.

She never could really understand my love for motorcycles
and the open road.
But she tried and a few times even went for a ride with me.

Sixty years. That's how long we were together.

   The Lois and Del love story started on a 25 degree below
zero night in 1954, in Fargo, North Dakota.

Love was certainly in the air that night, as it was the night
her journey through the abyss of Alzheimer's Disease came
to an end three weeks before our sixtieth anniversary.

2 - THE LOVE STORY OF LOIS AND DEL

In February 2014, 6 weeks before Lois passed away, I entered our story in the Helena Independent Record Valentines Day Love Story contest.
To my surprise we won. This is the story.

The Lois and Del Lonnquist love story began on Janury 25, 1954.
The Westernaires, a country band I was traveling with was booked into a club in Fargo, North Dakota. Severe weather made us late. It was 25 degrees below zero when we arrived. After playing the first 45 minute set I ran to a diner next door to get a hamburger.There coming to take my order was the most

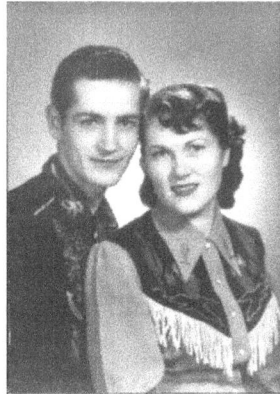

beautiful girl I had ever seen. The rest of the night, after each set I went to the diner. After midnight when we both finished work, I walked her home in the below zero cold. One week later I proposed. Three months later we were married. She was 18 years old and I was 19.
She played accordian I played guitar.
We performed as The Dakota Ramblers.
On our first anniversary we brought our first child home from the hospital. Five more children followed and we then performed as The Lonnquist Family Band.
Fifty Nine years and ten months have passed.
Alzheimer's Disease has stolen from her all the wonderful songs and memories. She no longer knows who I am.
But 60 years later I still know her as the most beautiful girl in the world and my love song for her will never end.

Lois passed away March 27, 2014
three weeks before our 60th Wedding Anniversary

3 - THE RIDE BEGINS

After the Memorial Service the kids asked, "What will you do now Dad?"
I said, "I think I'll go for a little ride."
That's how I came to be on the Interstate coming out of St. Louis, Missouri when the young guy hit the barrels of sand and lost control of his car.
No one was hurt in the mishap, but four lanes of cars and trucks were lined up for miles behind the accident scene.

Since I was blocking lane four I pulled the rig away from the concrete barrier and was soon on my way. Only now there was no traffic ahead of me and very little behind me. I was alone on the road and alone with my thoughts.

That's when I thought again about Lois, and what her reaction would have been and about those sixty years so full of memories. These last three years we cared for her at home. The kids and I.
I always liked to volunteer for groups like AARP, the Talking Book Library where I read books and teaching highway safety for both motorcycle and automobile drivers. When the doctors said she had moderate to late stage Alzheimer's I stopped all that.
Many folks reminded us that for most people with any kind of dementia a Care Center or Nursing Home would be best for her and for me and the kids.
I would nod my head and say they were probably right, but I knew in my heart there was only one place for Lois and that was in her own home, with her own husband and her own family. She was always such a modest, private person, a great lady and I knew we could provide the life that was best for her. 15 months she had been in the hospice program. With the help of the hospice staff, and our six kids we worked it out.
The kids and the hospice people worried about me too, but together we managed.

The "little ride" I mentioned took me back through the Midwest where we had lived through the early years and where we raised the six children.
North Dakota, Minnesota, Wisconsin, Iowa, South Dakota and Wyoming were included in that first 3,500 mile ride.
One day, when her decline into the abyss first began, I was riding through town when a guy in a pick up truck pulled out in front of me.
I had to lay the bike down to avoid a crash.
I wasn't hurt, but as I stood up all I could think of was, "What if I had broken a leg, I wouldn't be able to care for her, she would have to go to a nursing home or care center."
The vows we had taken sixty years earlier said I would be there for her in sickness or in health.
Those weren't just words. They were promises we had made to one another and she had taken care of me through two open heart surgeries and that accident where I fell off the roof and shattered my leg from the knee to the hip.
She was there for me, night and day for months each time.
I rode home, parked it, and quit riding motorcycles.

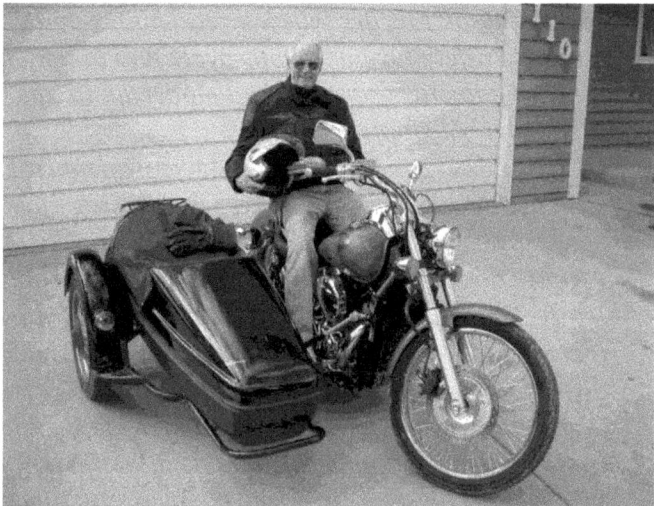

A few weeks later a friend called and said, "Del, you don't have to quit riding, put a sidecar on the bike."
And that's what I did.
The sidecar gave me a little more stability and I felt I could ride again, and still be the full time care giver I had promised I would be. That's why I was riding a rig with a sidecar when I had that little adventure near St. Louis. But that incident was in the spring, when I was on the way home from the long winter ride.

The Longest Ride started much earlier when my daughter Diana called from her home near Orlando, Florida and said, "Dad, why don't you leave Montana for awhile and spend the winter with us where it's warm and you can ride all winter?"
What a great idea. Out of the cold, into the land of sunshine. I thought this could be a great way to keep riding through the winter months. With daughters living in Orlando, Florida, Houston, Texas and San Jose, California, winter rides didn't seem nearly as daunting.
Planning for the ride began in earnest following the Memorial Service. Although she had passed away at the end of March, we postponed the service until June so kids and grandkids from all over the country and the world could plan for the trip to Montana.

The first night I met Lois I walked her home from her job as a waitress in a small diner and she had taught me the words and harmony to an old gospel song called, This World Is Not My Home.
We sang Gospel music together for the next sixty years, at first by ourselves and later, as the kids grew, in what we called the Lonnquist Family Band.
We decided it would be appropriate to have the family sing a gospel tribute to her as part of the Memorial Service.
Fifty Nine family members gathered in the church that June day to sing thirty minutes of her favorite music. It was a grand service, and one that is still talked about by those who were there.

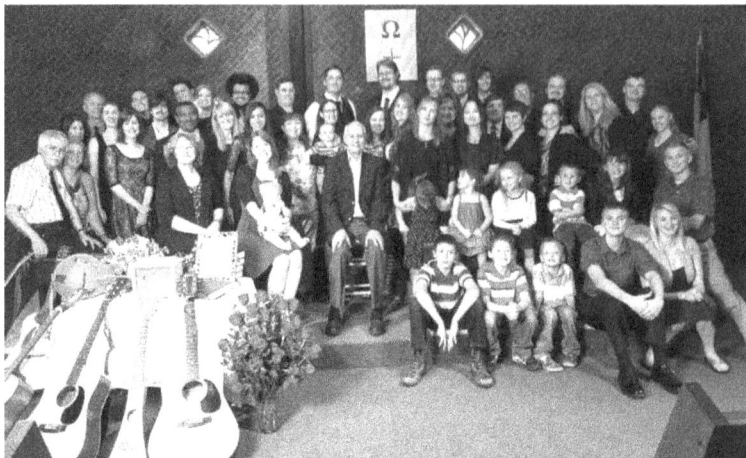

59 Family Members Sang Gospel Music for Lois
at First Lutheran Church in Helena, MT

Planning for The Ride, as I began calling it, needed to be extensive, and needed to fit a minimal budget.
Motels would be the biggest single expense and I began checking alternatives.

I found the best one at a place called Open Road Outfitters in Herndon, Virginia.
On their web site they showed videos of the Mini Mate tent camper which could be pulled behind a motorcycle.
The videos showed how it could be set up in two minutes and provide a bed six foot four inches in length and forty two inches wide, while weighing in at only 265 pounds.

I planned the trip to stop first in Minneapolis, Minnesota, and then to Baltimore, Maryland where I could visit Grandson Jason and his wife Allison.
Herndon would be only a few miles from there so I could visit and pick up the Mini Mate at the same time.

While checking mileage to Minneapolis I discovered it was exactly 1,044 miles to Monticello, Minnesota where my twin brother lived.

That's when the light went on.

I had thought for years about trying to become a member of a group dedicated to safe long distance motorcycle riding. The caveat to becoming a member of The Iron Butt Association, is that you have to ride 1,000 miles or more in a 24 hour period to earn your membership.

The Saddle Sore 1000 -1, it's called.

Planning and documentation had to be meticulous. Along with a Start of Ride Witness form and an End of Ride Witness form, I would have to save every gas receipt along the way and turn them in to the accreditation committee to prove I had met all of the requirements.

I had thought about that thousand mile ride in the past, but this was my opportunity.

4 - THE IRON BUTT CHALLENGE - SADDLESORE 1000-1

I started the ride at 4 AM in Helena, Montana with Barry Reddick of Helena as my Start of Ride Witness and Bill Ryder giving my machine a final check. Son Roger was there to take pictures.

Light rain was falling as I left the Helena truck stop service center where I had refueled and it continued for the first 90 miles of the ride, only changing to snow as I topped Bozeman Pass on I-90 two hours later.

The snow shower was brief and when I topped the pass and started down the east side it tapered off all together.

Three hours later the sun was shining and the wet riding gear began to dry out.

The mountains were soon behind me and I rolled out across the prairies of eastern Montana.

This was Lois' country.

She had grown up on a ranch in eastern Montana.

Although my career in broadcasting took us to many cities in many states, her heart was back home on the range.

She wrote a song about life on the ranch and that's what she called it:

"Back Home On The Range For Me."

We had wild roses in June and a Big Sky moon,
Cactus flower, sagebrush, and sweet pea
The Meadow Larks would sing
and the Bluebells would ring
Back Home on the Range for me.

As I raced by the Interstate mile markers, they were reminders of the distance I was traveling, and brought back memories of the markers that we had seen during Lois' physical and mental decline while making her own journey through this insidious disease called Alzheimer's.

It was in late November of 2011 when she came to the door of her office and asked me to dial our daughter Janis' number into her cell phone.

*She said the kids numbers I had programmed in to the
speed dial on her phone wouldn't work anymore.
I checked the speed dial. It worked.
She had forgotten how to use it.
Before Thanksgiving I discovered thirty checks missing
from the check book.
She had written checks and had forgotten to write them
into the check register.*

*She had always done the family book keeping and when I
asked about the missing checks she grew angry and
accused me of snooping in the books and said I caused the
error by switching some of the bills to on line payments.*

*That's when I called our son Roger and daughter Linda
and asked them to meet me at Perkin's restaurant for lunch
and to get some ideas on what to do.*

*Now we knew something was wrong, but still had hopes
that it was because she was wearing a new hearing aid, or
that the Systemic Scleroderma she was being treated for
could be the cause.*

*But the markers kept coming.
One day when I was reading a book for the Montana
Talking Book Library, Linda took her shopping.
When she made a purchase, she asked Linda to write the
check saying she was having trouble with her glasses and
couldn't see to write.
The slide into this dark world was, like the Interstate mile
markers, moving faster and faster.*

Having a sidecar on the motorcycle cuts the mileage by
up to 25 percent and meant I had to stop every hundred
miles for fuel.
That was good because I needed to get off the bike to
stretch and walk around a bit anyway, but bad because I
had 24 hours and no more to complete the ride.
Could I do it was the question?
Gas stops on an endurance ride like the Saddle Sore 1000
were supposed to be of short duration, but at nearly every
stop someone would come over and ask about the sidecar.
I got to meet many nice people, but it did take time.

I carried several old issues of The Sidecarist, the official magazine of the United Sidecar Association, and handed them out to anyone who asked more than the usual number of questions.

Before the ride Fast Signs of Helena had made a sign for the back of the bike which said, "80 Year Old Iron Butt Challenge Rider - 1000 Miles in 24 Hours."

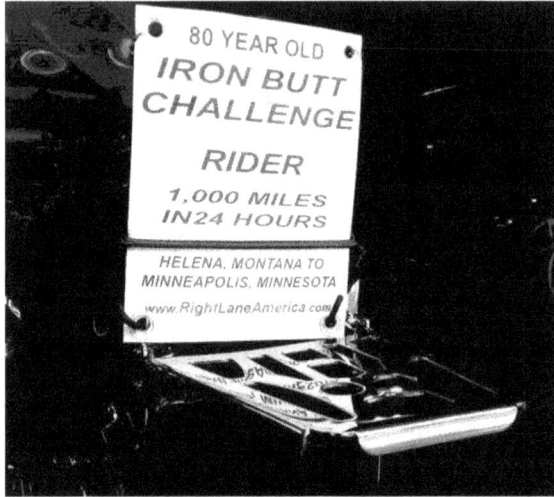

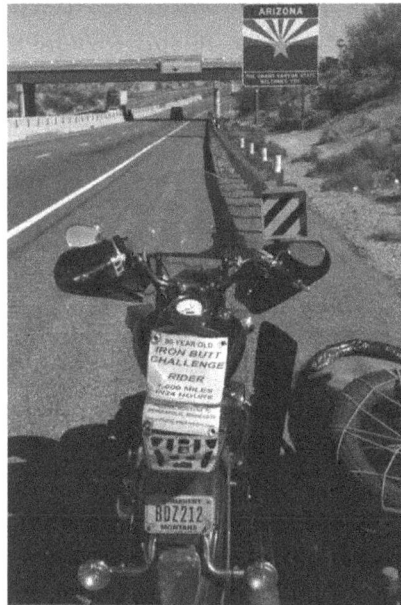

As I rode cars would come up behind me to pass and would then slow down as if to read the sign. The people in the cars and trucks would then smile as they drove by and give me a thumbs up as a show of support.

Oh, I know there were probably some who questioned why an 80 year old man would want to make such a trek, but my bike was ready, I was ready, and it would give me many hours in the saddle to think about, well, all of those things that I needed to think about.

It was a great ride.

Months later as I traveled through Houston, Texas a reporter from the Houston Chronicle asked that same question.

"Why did you want to make such a long endurance ride?"

I replied, "Because the kids and I traveled the long journey through Alzheimer's Disease together and we all needed to understand, there is life after Alzheimer's."

The Montana miles sped by and now I was nearing the North Dakota border, Lois' home area.

Here she had grown up riding Old Dixie, her favorite horse and playing with her sister Lucille and brother Stan in the Badlands which surrounded their home.

She had ridden the trails up hill and down, through rugged, snake infested country, always on the look out for the dangers that were inherent to the area.

Now she was riding an unfamiliar trail. One that was filled with even more dangers, but this insidious trail was all downhill with unknown dangers lurking before her every step.

Her first fall came on a day when I was once again narrating a book at the talking book library.

It was an unusually warm day in early December. She stepped out on the deck and her shoes got wet in the snow. When she walked through the kitchen the wet shoes slipped on the tile and down she went.

No serious injuries, but several bumps and bruises.

Alzheimer's Disease is a slippery slope that seems to wait for just the right moment to take you down.

One minute we would be having lunch and talking about the kids and grand kids and the next moment she would say, "I'm not hungry I think I'll go into my office and work for a little while."

Her office was her refuge.

Here she could sit by her desk and enjoy the peace that came with looking out over the Helena Valley and seeing the birds in the neighbors trees.

The computer was always on and she had the files from four years of research for her new book on the hard drive.

One day she said, "Del, this stupid computer is all messed up and I can't find my book files, I think I have deleted them for good."

There was desperation in her voice, losing the research files would be a real disaster.

I found the files for her and placed an Icon on the desktop so all she would have to do is click on it and the files would come up.

The relief that came with knowing the files were not lost was wonderful to see.

How hard it must be to have worked so hard on a project and then, unable to find the files on the computer, believe they are lost for good.

I went to Staples and purchased an external hard drive and saved all of the files on it.

A few days later she insisted I buy another external hard drive, in case the first one was stolen by burglars.

The paranoia that comes with Alzheimer's Disease and other forms of dementia was beginning to manifest itself. It was about this time that she began hiding things behind the clothes in the closets, behind the cans in the pantry and wherever she thought the burglars wouldn't find them.

The North Dakota border came and after a quick stop at the Painted Canyon Welcome Center, the one the kids always called The Buffalo Rest Area, because we saw buffalo there, I was back on the ride.

The sun had moved past it's zenith and I was trying to keep moving to get as many miles in as possible during the daylight hours so I would minimize the miles I would have to ride after dark.

North Dakota is known for long straight stretches of Interstate, even so, the land is not as flat as it seems and has long rolling hills which are much more noticeable when riding a motorcycle than they are when cruising through in a car.

The sidecar presented enough wind drag to slow the rig down and with a head wind or small incline it dragged even more.

This meant constantly adjusting the throttle lock, which is an inexpensive version of cruise control.

I was enjoying the wide open fields, some of which still carried remnants of the first good snowfall of the season. This is beautiful farm country and I have to admit I was enjoying the ride.

Bismarck, the state capital, was the half way point Lois and I always looked for when crossing the Dakotas.

We always stopped at a restaurant where they had a Mongolian stir fry.

A fun place, but one that I skipped on this trip as I moved past the city with only a quick stop for gas.

The cooler I carried in the sidecar was stocked with bottles of water and Ensure Nutrition drink as well as some Nature Valley Nutrition bars.

The rule for Long Distance, or LD riders, is no large meals. They make you tired and sleepy.

Snacks only is the rule, with lots of water to stay hydrated.

I was making good time and was mentally trying to calculate my arrival time.

I had left at 4 AM Mountain Time Saturday and would have to arrive in Monticello, Minnesota no later then 5 AM CDT Sunday morning to meet the 24 hour time limit for the ride.

I was on track to finish the ride at least two hours early, but could I maintain this steady pace after dark?

Half way between Bismarck and Fargo the shadows lengthened fast.
With a setting sun behind me I was now getting ready for the night ride.

Crossing the border into Minnesota the darkness was descending and headlights from a steady stream of westbound traffic reminded me of why I didn't like to ride or drive after dark.
Minnesota! Deer Country!
From Fargo to Monticello, through Fergus Falls, Alexandria, and the other cities, I didn't need the road side signs to remind me about the deer.

Years earlier I had hit a deer while riding and the broken collar bone kept me off the bike for many months.
Dreading this part of the ride I had installed a new LED extra bright headlight and this was my first chance to see what it would do.
It did not disappoint.
It lit up both lanes and the shoulders with such a brilliance that I could see almost twice as far down the road.
The darkness no longer posed a threat I couldn't handle.
I was looking forward to a celebration when the Saddle Sore 1000 -1 ride was completed, and I thought back to another celebration, the 75th anniversary of the Fort Peck Dam.

How honored Lois had felt when the Corps of Engineers asked her to take part in the dedication of a new memorial.

"Lois, Michele at the Fort Peck Interpretive Center needs you to make a decision about the 75th anniversary program of the Fort Peck Dam," I told her one morning.
"She has sent you another Email with questions about your speech and how much time you will need.
It was late January and they needed to plan their program.
While doing the research for her book Fifty Cents an Hour, Lois had found the names of fifty nine men who had been killed while working on the dam.

She had talked to Michelle many times about the lack of a memorial for these men. A memorial had been installed years earlier for the 8 men who died in the collapse of a portion of the dam during it's construction, but now she had the names of fifty nine men who died. One of them was her Father's best friend while they worked together on the 1930's construction project.

Because of her work in finding all of their names the Corps of Engineers had asked her to speak at the Dedication Ceremonies scheduled for June of 2012.

She had agreed to take part in the dedication and I sent an Email to Michelle telling her Lois would need about ten minutes for her part of the program.

At this point Lois was sure she could do the program and knew what she needed to do.

She was going to have a short speech and then she wanted me to join her for a song she had written about the workers and their families and the houses they lived in.

As the date of the program drew nearer and she hadn't written her speech I mentioned it to her several times. She reminded me that she had done many programs and didn't need my help in preparing for this one.

Two weeks before the event I wrote a short speech and included the song she had written.

The day before the dedication we drove to Glasgow, Montana and checked into the Cottonwood Inn where we always stayed on our trips to the dam.

Shortly after arriving she complained of feeling dizzy and lay down on the bed.

By evening she was pacing the room and talking about how she just wasn't up to doing the program and wanted to call Michelle and tell her she couldn't do it.

I suggested that she relax and not think about it and that if she wasn't feeling better by morning I could read her speech for her at the ceremony.

No sleep that night. She was disturbed and seemed to be having some kind of psychotic episode.

Knowing how important the dedication was to her and how Michelle was counting on her, at midnight I sat down and rewrote her talk so I could give it for her.

Neither one of us slept at all, the night was long and her medications didn't help calm her down.

In the morning it was worse and I explained to her that I would go to the dam site, fourteen miles away, and give the speech and asked her to promise that she would lay down and take a nap while I was gone.

The dedication went well, I did her talk for her, explaining that she had become ill during the night, the song she wrote was well received and many people said they hoped she would feel better.

Two hours after leaving I returned to the motel and she was not in the room.

I checked at the desk and they said they had seen an older woman carrying a plastic bag walking through one of the corridors a short time earlier.

It took only a few minutes to find her as she was walking through the hallway carrying a plastic bag filled with clothing from our suitcase. To keep it from being stolen she packed the clothes into the plastic bag and carried it with her. She didn't know where she was and said the maids had come to clean the room and she thought she had to leave and then couldn't find her way back.

She was very confused and very upset.

We were scheduled to do a forty five minute program that afternoon at the Interpretive Center and I called the center and cancelled it.

I told Lois we were going home and she began to calm down.

Twenty minutes later as we drove down the street on our way out of town she said, "Do you know what I would like?"

I said, "No what would you like?"

She replied, "A chocolate milkshake from McDonalds."

A quick stop and moments later she had her shake and we were driving down Highway two on our way home.

It was as if a light switch had been thrown and everything was good again.

The transformation that came when the stress of the program disappeared, and when she knew for sure that we were on our way home was amazing to see.

The seven hour drive across Montana was a happy ride. She was back to normal and as natural as always.

MY BAD! I should have talked her out of agreeing to do the program.

As the cognitive abilities declined I should have seen what the stress would do to her and explained that to the corps of engineers staff.

They were a caring and helpful group and Lois thought of Michelle as a dear friend.

The two of them had shared many projects together.

After arriving home I called Roger and Linda and met with them to discuss the weekend.

Roger had attended the dedication and already knew that Lois wasn't able to take part.

We talked about the coming days, weeks and months and what we thought we could expect, but were at a loss.

When we asked health care people what to expect, the response was nearly always,

"Well, you know everyone is different, so it's hard to tell."

I attended an Alzheimer's support group but was the only one who came. No help there. Pamphlets and books were suggested, but practical, down to earth help was sparse and hard to find.

It seems all of the research being done was aimed at the early stages of the disease and moderate and late stage help was not readily available. Health care people are caring and friendly but being a care giver, oftentimes, seemed to be a do it yourself project.

Thank Heaven for the kids.

They were the support group that made home care possible.

I was in the last lap of my thousand mile ride.
Central Minnesota deer country and I was watching the
highway shoulders for both deer and pieces of truck tires.
There was no moon.

The bright new headlight did what it was supposed to do
while on bright, but with an unending stream of traffic
headed in the opposite direction, I was unable to use the
light on bright for any extended period.
No matter, I was ahead of schedule and moving steadily
toward my goal.
Watching for deer was one thing, but the real danger
seemed to be from large pieces of truck tires which
appeared frequently on the shoulder of the road and
sometimes in the driving lane.
They were hard to see against the dark asphalt and required
close attention.
Hitting one small piece of tire tread would put a quick end
to my endurance ride.
I gave all of my attention to the road ahead.

*The same close attention I tried to maintain while
spending my days with Lois and the many unexpected
things she would do.*

*There never seemed to be a reason for her sudden urge to
begin walking quickly from one room to another, as if
searching for something but unable to remember exactly
what it was she was looking to find.*
*These sudden urges to wander brought us to the realization
that we needed to do more for security.*
*Children's locks on cupboard doors and alarms for
exterior doors.*
*I placed a lock on the closet doors too, but she pulled on
the door until the lock snapped off.*
It made her laugh.
*Did she laugh because she knew she had out witted those
who would try and control her environment, or was it
something else that delighted her?*
We would never know.

About that time we tried Christmas shopping but one trip through the toy section was too much and she said, "I want to go home, it's too noisy and I need time to think."
We later decided on Amazon Gift Certificates which we could order on line.
Grocery shopping was the same.
We did get some items into the cart but when we got to the checkout she was getting more and more confused by the noisy speakers and crowds of people.
I suggested she to go over by the door and sit on the bench and wait for me.
From then on I did the shopping without her.
Noisy speakers in the stores and the crowds of people seemed to disorient her and she would become increasingly apprehensive.
When I told her I was going shopping she would say, "I think I should go along so you don't forget anything.
I would say, "Great, get your coat and we'll do it together."
At that point, without fail she would change her mind and tell me about all of the things she had to get done around the house.
I tried to shop early since late afternoon and evening became harder for her to handle.

It was Linda who first told me about Sundown Syndrome that affected many people with various forms of dementia.
I learned that I was supposed to close the drapes before the sun began dropping down behind the mountains.
This brought some relief and if I turned up the Slack Key Guitar music provided by the Pandora music service, and got her settled down in her recliner, we could hold at bay the fears that coming darkness brought.
How hard these fears must have been for her.
I could hold her hand and talk with her, but the darkness that was slowly taking over her every thought and mood was always there, lurking close by, ready to pounce at the slightest interruption in her routine.

The lights of the Holiday Gas Station in Monticello, Minnesota were bright as I pulled off the Interstate ramp, down the street and up to their gas pumps.
I dismounted and looked at my watch.
1:50 AM CDT!   I MADE IT!
I made it with just over two hours to spare.

For over two and a half years Lois and I, with the help of our six children, had journeyed through a terrible disease called Alzheimer's. The journey had ended in March and now this remarkable family and I were proving to each other, that there was indeed, Life after Alzheimer's Disease.

The Iron Butt One Thousand Mile Ride, was an expression of faith.
Faith in a life still rich and full.
It was a great ride, one that I most certainly will do again.
I called my twin brother Dean and asked him to come to the station and sign my End-of-Ride witness form and then sent text messages to all six kids to let them know I had made it.
1,044 miles in under 22 hours!
I was an Iron Butt Rider.
The Iron Butt Association slogan is:
"Worlds Toughest Riders."
This was a license plate frame I would mount on the bike and an emblem that I would display with pride.
Tired? Not a bit. I was elated.
This was not a speed race. It was an endurance challenge and at the age of 80 I had prevailed.
It was a good feeling and one that brings a warm glow anytime I'm riding and another rider gives a friendly wave as they pass traveling in the other direction.

It's a fraternity, this group of men and women who have a passion for riding a motorcycle and it is almost impossible to convey this passion to a non-rider with mere words.
I'm one of them!
IBA number 60280.
Out of the millions of riders world wide, I am one of 60,000 who have made *the ride*.

Oh sure, most of the other members of the IBA have ridden many of these thousand mile and longer endurance rides, but the first one will always be the one I will remember. I salute the more than sixty thousand riders who are members of this close knit fraternity.
Salute!

5 - MINNEAPOLIS TO BALTIMORE

After a good days sleep at Dean's house and a dinner out with Dean, his wife Bev, my sister Vivian and her husband Dave, I set off on the next leg of the trip.
This time through Mankato, Minnesota where I stopped at Bethany College to take Grand Daughter Lydia out for a motorcycle ride and a pizza.
It was a good visit and I then began the ride south through Iowa, Illinois, Indiana, Ohio, Pennsylvania and ultimately to Grandson Jason and Allison's house in Maryland.

Riding the farm country highways through Iowa and Indiana gave me hours to think about the life we had shared for all of those years.

I remembered Pastor Miller saying after the Memorial Service "Del, you have a great family."
I said, "It was easy, all I had to do was marry a great lady."
She was a great Mother to our six kids.
Sewing special clothing for all of the special occasions, and the outfits we all wore when we were performing as the Family Band.

One of the kids had said, "I just can't imagine how she found time to do all of that sewing, with all of the other things she was doing in those busy years."

She had been a reporter, photographer, music teacher, writer of songs, author and more, but most of all she had been a Wife, Mother, Grand Mother and Great Grand Mother.

Her book, Fifty Cents An Hour, The Builders and Boomtowns of the Fort Peck Dam, had been a good seller for historical societies around the state and even nationwide.
That's what made the speed of her decline so hard to get my head around.

Although there had been signs of forgetfulness, it was easy to blame it on her hearing problem or the Systemic Scleroderma she had been diagnosed with years earlier.

Alzheimer's Disease was something old people get and we were only in our mid 70's.

The day I discovered this meticulous household and business bookkeeper had written 30 checks that were not written into the check register I knew something was seriously wrong.

Yet, she could carry on a great conversation on the phone with the kids who lived far off in other states, and could hold her own in Wii Bowling which we did on Monday nights following Antique Road Show on PBS. It was her favorite show.

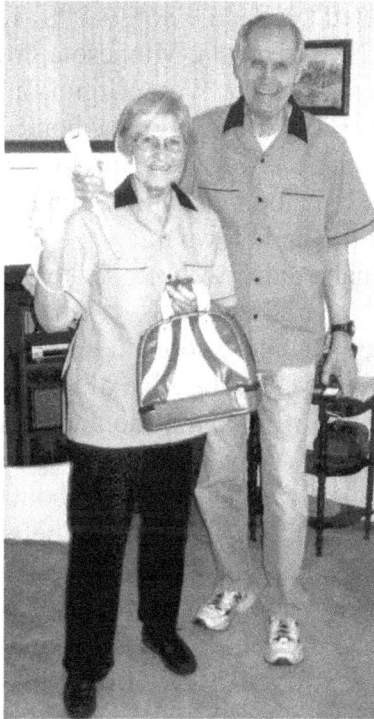

Janis and Mike had sent us Bowling Shirts and a bowling ball bag to carry the Wii bowling system in.
The Wii Bowling was good exercise until one night she just couldn't seem to remember when to let go of the trigger that let the ball go down the alley.

We switched to Dominos and had some great Monday night Domino games.

Then came the night when she pushed her left over pieces to Linda and said, "Can you count the spots, I just can't see them very good tonight."
As others who have traveled the Alzheimer's journey know, it seems to sneak up on you and all of a sudden, when you least expect it, this insidious disease will pounce on you and steal away memories and life's great experiences.
This it did to Lois who was so loved by us all.

It was all going so well.
I completed the Saddle Sore 1,000 -1, and made the run through North Dakota, Minnesota, Iowa, Illinois, Indiana, Ohio, Pennsylvania, West Virginia and into Maryland.
Less then 100 miles from the home of Grandson Jason, I was cruising up I-68 at 65 MPH when I heard a loud bang, followed by a loud whistling sound.
The rear tire had blown out.
The Yamaha didn't wobble, shake or swerve.
It stayed as solid as a rock.
A tribute to the great job Bill Ryder did in setting it up.
I quickly moved to the edge of this very busy freeway and pulled as far off onto the shoulder as I could.
I have Triple A Premium covering motorcycle tows, thanks to son Roger telling me about this AAA add on.
I got the Triple A card out, but before I could make the call, a sharp looking Harley Davidson Sportster pulled over and it's rider sporting a beard, leather jacket and denim vest covered with patches from Biker get-togethers around the country got off and asked if I needed help.
"Blew the rear tire" I said.
Without waiting Sportster guy, Dave Brode said " that's not a good deal let me make a couple of calls."
Minutes later he had located a tire at Twigg's Cycles in Hagerstown, some forty miles away and scheduled me in for as soon as we could get there.
I got the Triple A card out and tried to call for a tow truck.

With all of the trucks roaring past I couldn't hear well enough to get Triple A for a tow truck.

Just then one of Dave's friends pulled up in his SUV. Seeing that I was having trouble with my call he told me to get in his car, away from the highway noise.

Triple A was fast in lining up a towing service to haul me the forty miles into town.

They said it would be an hour to get the truck .

Much to my surprise, in less that five minutes I received a call from Scott Carbough owner/operator of Jaz's Towing and Recovery service of Hancock, Maryland.

He wanted to confirm the location I was at.

I told him I was on I-68 East near Exit number 68.

Dave had pinpointed the location for me when he first arrived on the scene.

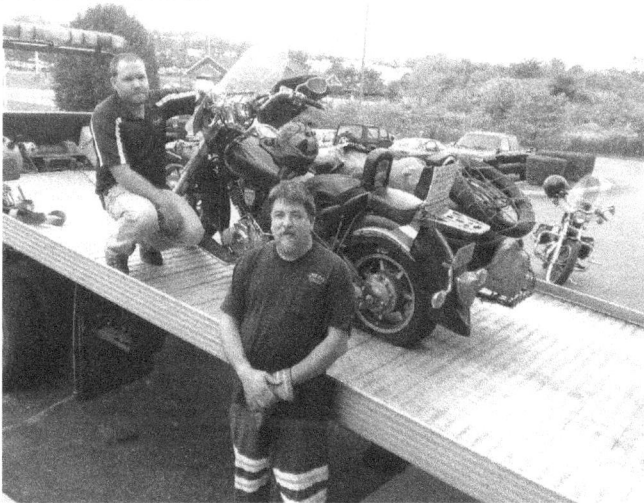

Service Advisor Andy Horowitz & Scott Carbough
Twigg's Cycle Shop in Hagerstown, MD

To my surprise Scott said he was already at Exit 68 but in the West bound lane.

When he received the call from Triple A, he had been on the way to a relatives house to check on some needed repairs on his truck.

His Uncle lived close to the spot where I was stranded. Instead of an hour long wait for the truck, he was there in a matter of minutes.

In a short time he had my rig loaded on his truck and 45 minutes later he was backing up to the loading dock at Twiggs Cycles in Hagerstown, the largest motorcycle shop in the area.

Service Advisor Andy Horowitz quickly had the bike moved into the shop and the crew went to work.

As Harley Sportster Dave put it, " I think God was working overtime to get you taken care of today, if your tire had blown a half mile further down the road you would have had no cell phone service, it's a dead zone for cell phones."

Yeah, I think he got it right.

On this day, all the good came together for me.

Life is good.

I had a great ride today and a very interesting afternoon. Met new friends and have another good story to share at side car rallies and other get-togethers.

That's what Lois would have said too: "Your Guardian Angel was watching out for you when that tire blew out." She would have been right.

She always seemed to know just the right thing to say when something happened. It was hard to see that quick thinking and repartee slowly fade away.

But the fading memory did bring some humorous moments too.

One morning Linda was helping her with her bath when she looked up and said, "Is Linda coming today?"

It was a sudden reminder that the decline in what the doctors called "cognitive ability" was continuing it's slow, steady advance and it startled Linda.

A short time later we were sitting at the dining room table having coffee when she stood up to leave the table. I said, "Where are you going Lois?" She replied, "I'm going on a date with my new boy friend."

I looked at Linda and said, "Well, I think leaving for a date with a new boy friend trumps is Linda coming today."

It was a humorous but sad moment, and showed again the extent of the decline and how quickly things were changing. What were we to do about it. That was the question.
And this was a question with no immediate answer until our daughter Diana called with an idea.

She had been checking on a disease called Normal Pressure Hydrocephalus which brought a rapid decline in memory. She thought that since her Moms decline had come on so quickly it might not be Alzheimer's Disease after all.
Linda had also read a report on it.

Diana wanted to schedule Mom into a Florida clinic that specialized in dementia, in all of it's forms.

We began plans for a flight to Florida and with some hope scheduled the appointment.

After the blown tire incident I rode another fifty miles and with a light rain falling I found a motel and had a good nights sleep.

The next morning I got an early start, planning on arriving in the big city of Baltimore during the early Saturday morning hours when traffic would be light.
I arrived in Brooklyn, Maryland for my visit with Jason and Allison with no further problems. It was Saturday and Grand daughter Crystal and her husband Ryan came from New York to spend the day with us.

Jason took us all to Fort McHenry which turned out to be a fascinating place to visit. Especially since only a few weeks before PBS had shown a special on the Star Spangled Banner and part of the program centered on Fort McHenry and was live from the place we were visiting.

Sunday morning was special as I attended church with them and Jason led the Praise Band at the North Arundel Church. We shared a family joke after church about how this family praised the Lord from Coast to Coast, since another Grandson, Vaughn leads the Praise Band at Apostle's Lutheran Church in San Jose, California.

Monday morning at 7 AM, we headed for Open Road Outfitter's in Herndon, VA to pick up my Mini Mate tent trailer.

Jason took the day off and led me through the Washington DC traffic.

It was a great feeling, climbing on the Yamaha and looking back to see my new Tent Camper following up the street.

It hadn't taken Dale Coyner long to hook up the trailer hitch and lighting harness. As I was getting ready to leave Dale handed me a signed copy of his book, Motorcycle Journeys Through North America .

It was well used throughout the rest of my 16,000 mile trek.

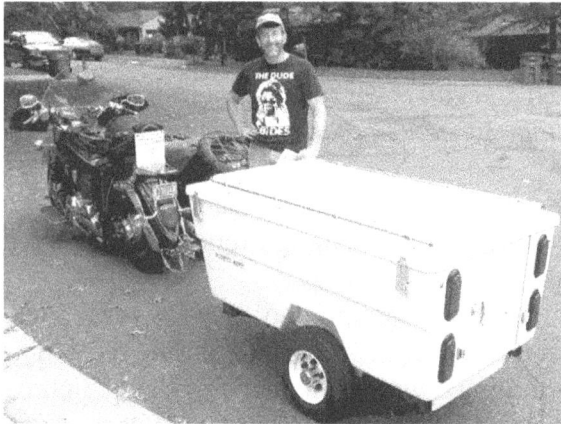

Dale Coyner - Open Road Outfitters

The trek we made to the Dementia Clinic in Florida was often on my mind. We had fears of what would happen if she became frightened or upset, or if the crowded plane would be a problem. As I think about it now I realize we were very fortunate.

The flight to Florida went better than we expected thanks to Linda flying with us. Janice and Roger also made a special photo album that kept Lois busy and her great comfort.

The day went well. Diana and Ilidio were waiting for us at the airport.

The next week we met with a team of 10 doctors and nurses who had been reading through the twelve years of medical records they had requested in advance.

We had gathered records from every doctor and hospital she had been treated at and now the team was ready to meet Lois and ask her the questions that would give them the final pieces of information they would need.

They used a simple two page list of questions, i.e." can you tell us what year it is, can you draw a clock and show the time is 3 PM" and some that she had previously been asked by doctors in Helena.

Following this meeting they asked for lab tests and set up another appointment in a month.

It was a long month as we waited for them to plow through all of the information and test results.

Meanwhile Lois had a lot of attention from Diana, Ilidio and many visitors. She spent hours walking through the garden and had amazing clarity on some days and also days of tears.

She managed to work the lock on the gate and went for a walk down the street on one occasion, while everyone scattered through the neighborhood trying to find her.

She was tired but unharmed when they found her and brought her home in the car.

She responded well each evening to the poems and stories that Diana read and slept well.

Finally came the day we looked forward to and dreaded at the same time. The Team was ready with their findings. The team was made up of friendly, caring health care professionals who treated both Lois and the family members with kindness, but that didn't make it any easier to accept their report.

She did not have Normal Pressure Hydrocephalus. The senior doctor said we have determined that she has moderate to late stage Alzheimer's Disease.

I asked, "How did you reach that conclusion?"
The doctor replied, "We just eliminated everything else. There is no question that this is Alzheimer's."

He confided in me after the meeting that it was probably closer to late stage than moderate.
We rented a car to drive Lois back to Montana.

6 - THE MINI MATE TENT TRAILER

The new Mini Mate tent camper was no problem as it pulled smoothly and evenly behind the Yamaha.
People had warned me about the trailer swaying back and forth, but it never happened.
It was easy to forget the trailer was there.
I checked the mirrors often and it never moved off the straight line it was following.
The kids would be happy to hear about that. I knew some of them would be worried.

I found a McDonald's Restaurant where I could have lunch and use their WiFi to bring the Face Book group, "Where In The World Is Grandpa" up to date.
The kids and grandkids said they looked forward to the twice daily updates so they would know where I was and that I was doing okay.

A Face Book message from Grand daughter Lorna was waiting for me as I checked in. A reminder that when I reached Florida I was to schedule time for a cruise.
Her husband Rosario was First Officer on a cruise ship and they had an eight day cruise planned.

As I returned a message I remembered the day Lois came running out of her office calling out, "Del, Del the cruise ship is sinking and Lorna and the kids are on it!"

She was very distressed, wide eyed and in tears as she thought her grand daughter and great grand children were in danger.

I went into her office and we listened as the news of the sinking of the Costa Contra cruise ship in Italy was being reported on all the news channels.

She had the Disney Cruise ship that Lorna was on confused with the Costa Contra.

She was terrified and it was a long time before she understood what I was trying to explain, that it was a different cruise ship and that all her children were safe. Fear, panic and paranoia feelings seemed to be coming with increasing frequency.

She would hear a news story from overseas and confuse it with what was happening to us.

The city sanitation truck would bang the garbage cans and she would rush to the window to see who was trying to break in to the house.

These were real fears and in her troubled mind they all seemed to mix together.

How frightening this must have been for her as she hid jewelry, musical instruments and the CD's containing the files for her new book under the bed, in the closet and in a chest of drawers.

It was a fearful time that often brought her to tears.

As I left McD's I typed the GPS coordinates Dale gave me into my smart phone and the Verizon Navigator took me to Front Royal, Virginia and on to Skyline Drive. Skyline Drive winds through The Shenandoah National Park and ends at the beginning of the Blue Ridge Parkway.

I stopped at Mathews Arm Camping Site and used my National Park Golden Passport to save 50% on the $15.00 camping fee. The Golden Passport had been a purchase Lois and I made many years ago for future National Park and Historic site use. It has paid for itself over and over again through the years.

It was just beginning to rain as I, for the first time, followed the directions for setting up the Mini Mate Tent camper. It was easy and took only slightly longer than the two minutes I had previewed on-line.

It was only 5:30 PM, but already getting dark as the storm clouds moved in.

By 6:30 PM, the wind was howling and it continued unabated until near dawn.

The rain fell very hard and the wind seemed to roll over the camp in waves. Slacking off for a few minutes and then coming back with renewed fury.

The storm which the next day rolled through Maine
dropping trees and power lines, now, in the mountains,
lashed out at a novice camper, while he wondered if his
newly purchased Mini Mate was up to the challenge.
It Was!

Although the tent sides billowed inward slightly, the
trailer itself didn't budge.
The legs held it firmly in place.
Opening the tent flaps at dawn showed the rain and wind
were gone.

Now only a cold breeze brought a chill to the morning
and breaking down the camp site was a short job,
completed with sweater, coat, hat and gloves on.

The day warmed quickly and by early afternoon I had
reached the end of Skyline Drive.
I looked at the map of the Blue Ridge Parkway and
wondered if I was up to riding four hundred more miles of
the winding, twisting roadway.

My arms and shoulders were definitely showing the
effects of driving a sidecar rig through the rugged country.
It's not like riding a two wheeler through the twisties.

As I was debating whether to head for I-95 and Florida, a
text from Diana set my course.
She told of an air show at Daytona Beach this weekend and
how we could camp on the beach.
Florida sunshine sure sounded better than another cold
night in the mountains.
I turned left onto I-64 and headed for I-95 and Florida.
The Mini Mate, the all night wind and rain storm, and the
Skyline Drive made for a great adventure.

A new adventure awaited my arrival in Lake Mary, Florida.

Storms like the one in the Shenandoah National Forest brought great fear and dread to Lois. She would rush to the window if lightening flashed or thunder rumbled in the night.

She was constantly checking the doors to see if they were locked so burglars could not get in.

We installed an awning to cool the southwest facing deck and give her a place where she could be outside and yet we wouldn't have to worry about her wandering off.

But there was a day when she got out of the house and did wander off.

It happened while I was in the garage picking up pieces for the awning.

I left the big garage door in the raised position and had left the door between the kitchen and the garage slightly ajar.

While I was looking for what I needed for the awning, she slipped out the door and was gone down the street.

Moments later I discovered she was not inside and ran around the house looking for her.

She was nowhere to be found.

Now I was the one who was terrified.

I jumped in the car and raced down to the first corner.

Far down the street I saw a flash of pink, like the sweater she was wearing.

I turned and two blocks down the street found her lying in the gutter.

She had stepped off the curb and had fallen.

An older couple from an apartment complex across the street had already started over to help.

I turned around parked in the middle of the street.

Running to her I saw a scared, puzzled look on her face.

That's when the tears came.

With the help of the elderly couple I got her into the car and moments later was pulling in to our garage.

She was okay!

I was trembling at the thought that she might have been lost and I would be unable to find her.

We've all heard the stories on the news about how a dementia patient had wandered off and was lost.

This was the scariest moment we had experienced up to that point and sent me in to a flurry of activity looking for the perfect lock for exterior doors and berating myself for that one moment of carelessness that could have ended in disaster.

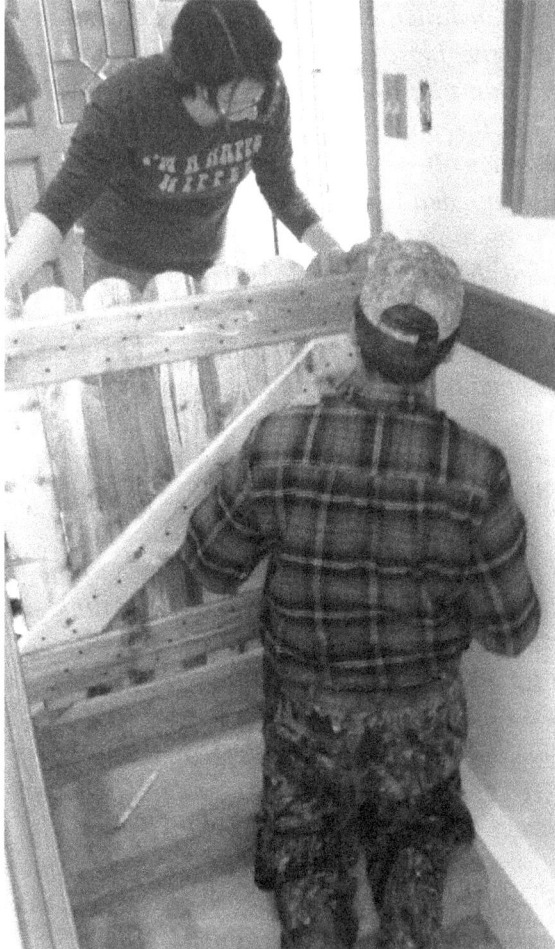

Hanna & Aaron

I researched locks and dementia aids on line.

The kids found door alarms that made a loud whistle when the door was opened.

If she managed to unlock the door the alarm would go off and it startled her. At first she would quickly close the door and say, "Those darn birds." She soon discovered that she could still go through the door, even if it was making the noise that sounded like birds.

Grandkids Hanna and Aaron made a heavy wooden locking gate for the stairway to the lower level..

It seemed that constant attention was the only solution that really worked.

As I made the turn off I-64 and on to I-95 south I relaxed and sat back to enjoy the sunshine and the ride.

The ride was thing.

Enjoy the ride, was what I had told so many students through the years.

It's not just a ride. It's an experience.

The trailer followed smoothly with little or no effect on the Yamaha.

From 25 MPH to 75 MPH it was flawless.

Travel was smooth, not like the winding twisting roads of the Skyline Drive.

The Interstate made for an easy ride.

The sign on the back of the Yamaha read:

80 Year Old Iron Butt Challenge Rider
1000 miles in 24 hours.

I had made good use of the sign when I missed the 270 cut off around Columbus, Ohio.

I drove right through downtown Columbus and through the evening rush hour traffic on I-70.

On several occasions when I got in the wrong lane I would put on my turn signals, look back and people would see the sign and wave me into the right lane.

Columbus, Ohio has lot's of friendly people and they treated an old biker very kindly.

I tried to maintain a 65 mile per hour pace as I cruised down the interstate where most traffic was moving at 70 MPH or more.

People in passing cars would read the sign and give me a thumbs up, wave, or in many cases slow down long enough to shoot a picture with their cell phone camera. It must have been the most photographed sign on the highway.

In Iowa a young father with three sons in his car whizzed up along side then slowed quickly and pulled in behind so they could take pictures. Pulling alongside they all smiled, waved and gave the thumbs up.

This became a familiar sight as people young and old laughed, waved, smiled and gave the thumbs up salute. The old motorcycle rider safety adage that you go where you are looking proved true on several occasions as people intent on reading the sign slowly drifted over the center line into my lane.

In South Carolina a young lady was so intent on getting a good picture that as she drifted into my lane I was forced to cross the rumble strip onto the shoulder of the road. She was shocked and embarrassed when she discovered what she had done, but a smile and a wave from me brought a similar response from her.

At gas stations, rest areas and food stops fellow travelers would go out of their way and take the time to say how good it was to see an older person doing something special like the SaddleSore 1000-1 of the Iron Butt Association.

What would seem a joke at first took on a more serious note when I explained that the organization promoted safe long distance motorcycle touring.

It began to dawn on me that age, race, ethnicity and belief didn't seem to matter.
Most Americans really do love, honor and respect older people and show those feelings in many ways.

Since leaving Helena, Montana on September 27th, I have traveled thousands of miles across the United States.
Through the evening rush hour traffic in Columbus, Ohio to the Monday morning rush hour traffic around Washington DC, people were kind and courteous.

What a great experience.

Through Montana, Idaho, North and South Dakota, Washington state, Wyoming, Minnesota, Wisconsin, Iowa, Illinois, Indiana, Ohio, West Virginia, Virginia, Pennsylvania, Maryland, North and South Carolina, Georgia and Florida people have been fantastic .

Thank You America for your scenic beauty and for your multitudes of great people.

People who wave, smile and support an 80 year old man in his quest to ride across the country on his motorcycle. From bikers to truck drivers American travelers had expressed their support for this ride in so many ways.

The word I heard the most at truck stops and rest areas was "Inspiration."

As if to say other older citizens might be prompted to live out their dreams and take another look at the proverbial Bucket List.

The most frequent question I have received is, "Are you really traveling all by yourself."

I got the feeling the deeper question they were asking was: "You mean your kids are letting you do this on your own?" I know this has not been easy for kids, but frequent updates on the Face Book group "Where In The World Is Grandpa" kept them up to date on the latest travels.

Another question heard frequently was, "Don't you have a radio to keep from getting bored?"

My response was, "As I travel I have a lifetime of memories which I can play back at will with no need for a navigation screen, Sirius XM, Bluetooth or GPS."

The memories are as bright and real today as when they were lived all those years ago.

Lois had memories too.
I would get her settled into the recliner where she slept now. She seemed to need the comfort of the chair arms on each side of her as if she felt safer and more secure.

I slept in my recliner too and moved it to a position directly opposite from hers so I could see her as she slept.
For many months she slept through the entire night.
Then suddenly, with no warning came the dark time when I would be awakened at 2 AM by low moaning and sobbing.
Nothing I could do or say seemed to help.
I would sit by her side, hold her hand and talk to her.
The crying would last up to an hour or so and then she would drop off into a fitful, uneasy sleep.
The nightmares continued for several months.
I would ask her what was frightening her, with no response.
   Then, one night, in the middle of the nightmare, she sobbed out the words, "I took the kids and hid under the kitchen table all night."
   There it was. During one of her Father's violent outbursts she had taken her younger brother, Stan and sister Lucille and hid under the table.
Growing up in an unstable, often violent home had given her some terrible things to remember.
Locked away in the deep recesses of her mind for the sixty years we were together and only now coming back to haunt her with these nightly visions.
   Roger's wife Janice said she had read about dementia patients who had regressed through their lifetimes and relived the good times and the bad times with their dreams. Lois had apparently been reliving those terrible childhood episodes in her nightmares. Terrible times that she had buried deep in her sub-conscious for all of those years.
Months later they stopped as suddenly as they had begun.

   Came the night when she slept through until morning and awoke looking more rested and at ease then had been the case for many months.
What an insidious disease this Alzheimer's is.
First your memory begins to slip away and you can't remember the things you have always done so easily every day and then without warning the terrible things you don't want to remember come flooding back to haunt you.

This had been a hard time.
It was very difficult to hear the sobbing and crying
night after night, unable to do anything to soothe her.
How good it was when those unhappy memories had run
their course and she could once again enjoy a deep,
untroubled sleep.

My second night of camping in the tent camper was at a
KOA campgrounds on the south side of Savanah, Georgia.
It was a good warm night, unlike the National Forest camp
in the mountains.
The sun was shining with temperature in the 70's as I was
setting up the camp.
The tent material was still wet from the night before but
dried quickly in the bright sun.
It was a quiet night.
I woke up early and was soon on the road heading for Lake
Mary, Florida, where family was waiting.
From Savanah it was an easy drive down I-95 and I-4 to
Lake Mary and the GPS described each turn I was
supposed to make.
By early afternoon I pulled into the Sacramento driveway.
I had ridden 3,600 miles.
From Helena, Montana to Lake Mary, Florida.
How good it was to settle back in a lounge chair on the
lanai and soak in the sun.
Life is good.

7 - KEY WEST
THE SOUTHERMOST POINT IN THE USA

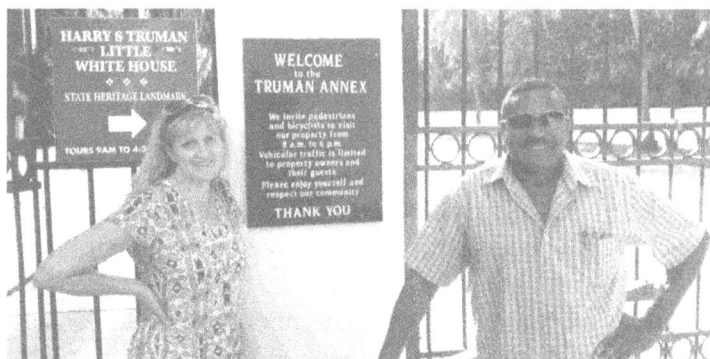

Diana and Ilidio at the
Truman Little White House

Diana and Ilidio maintain an interesting and fun life style, with numerous friends and relatives dropping in on an almost daily basis.

Makes for a warm friendly, welcoming atmosphere and one that I rapidly began to enjoy.

Morning coffee in the sunshine on the lanai, short rides around town and planning for the next adventure.

It came quicker then I had expected.

Diana wanted me to make the ride to Key West, the southernmost point in the USA.

They would drive the car with their camping equipment and I would ride the bike and pull the tent camper behind.

This sounded like a great trip.

Friends Americo and Angela living in Miami would be the stop over at the halfway point where we could get a good nights rest as well as a good visit with their friends. I even took Angela for a ride in the sidecar.

From Miami we would make the run down to Key West and see the sights. The ride was fantastic with ever longer bridges between the keys with the Atlantic Ocean on one side and the Gulf of Mexico on the other. Colorful sails from a hundred sail boats on both sides of the highway.

At each gas or rest stop other travelers would come over and inquire about the sidecar and camping trailer.
Some gave me business cards and invited me to visit if I ever rode into their area.

Diana had researched on line to find interesting places to visit and high on the best places list was the President Harry Truman Little White house.
The guide, who even looked a little like the former president, gave a lively tour.
The next stop was to get a picture of me on the Yamaha riding by the sign saying "This is the Southernmost Point In The USA - 90 miles to Cuba."

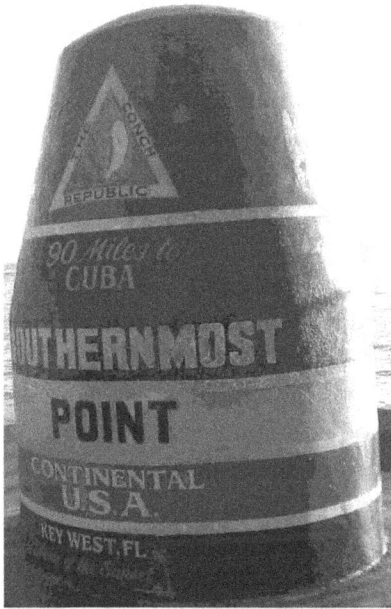

There was a long line of people waiting to get their picture standing by the sign. This was a popular tourist stop and all around us people were laughing and obviously enjoying their visit to Key West.

I rode slowly by the sign while Diana shot a video and people watched with amusement as the old biker with the sidehack and trailer rode slowly past.
We were indeed the quintessential tourists.

As I parked the rig after riding past the southernmost sign a young couple came running across the street.
The young man was shouting, "Mister, Mister, I must shake your hand! I must shake your hand!"

From Puerto Rico, now living in Tampa, they had passed us on the way down to Key West, slowed so they could read the sign, then laughing and waving, had ridden on past, only to spot the rig again as I rode by the sign.

What a nice young couple, he on a Harley Sportster and she riding a pink Honda.

How cool for them to come to where I was parking to shake hands and visit.

People are so great.

After a cool evening ride from Key West we arrived at the Bahia Honda Florida State Campground.

We pulled into the parking spot an hour after dark.

In a few minutes I was all set up and sitting at the picnic table with a glass of wine while Diana and Ilidio struggled with their tent poles.

I did have to chuckle as they put up the tent which took so much longer than my little Mini Mate.

While sitting by the table I heard a rustling noise behind me and as I turned to look Diana shouted, "Raccoon."

The wily little rascal had jumped up on the table, snared a bag of potato chips and was gone into the brush before anyone could make a move to get him. The cheeky little devil found a large nearby bush to hide under and crunched the chips loudly, as if to rub salt in the wound.

Ilidio's campfire chicken was great and the sound of nearby ocean waves made sleep come quickly.

The next day brought a beautiful ride which carried us back to our Miami friends house. There we shared more visiting, more good food and another good nights sleep.

Next day we found bright sunshine and a fantastic ride through a beautiful part of Florida.

As we approached Orlando the sunshine disappeared and dark clouds moved in. With traffic heavy I couldn't stop to put on my wet weather riding gear.

In a matter of minutes the rain became a downpour and I was soaked to the skin. Riding in the rain while soaked is not bad when the weather is warm so it was still a nice ride.

At one point while going over one of the many Interstate over/underpasses I saw brake lights on a vehicle in front of me and touched my brakes.

The wet roadway, the brakes, the sidecar, all joined together to send me spinning sideways out of control.

I ended up sliding into the next lane and while skidding sideways went right on past Diana and Ilidio in their car.

It wasn't a dangerous skid, just a wet road and a slide out. As I approached their car all I could think of was, "Oh no I'm going to scratch Diana's new car."
I didn't scratch it though and as Ilidio pulled ahead of me we were once again on our way home, with one more small adventure behind us.

What a great trip to Key West, Florida, the southernmost point of the USA.

The next day while seated on the lanai with my morning coffee I thought about the friends I had made on our trek to Key West, and I remembered the many people who joined Lois and I in our Alzheimer's journey.

The friends from Frontier Hospice helped the family and I through the illness which seemed to stretch out much longer then anyone expected.

The wonderful bath lady came on Tuesday and Friday mornings to help Lois in her bath, gently helping her walk from her recliner to the bathroom.

Linda, worked nights as an RN at the VA Hospital and had been doing the bath after she got off work three mornings a week. Having the bath lady come to help Lois with her bath was a great blessing for Lois and it took a great load off Linda's shoulders. What a great service it was. Even with the use of a bath bench which she could sit on during her bath it became increasingly difficult to make the move from recliner to the bathtub. Then came the morning when the bath lady reminded me that the hospital bed we had recently ordered and which was in the living room, but not being used, would soon be needed as Lois' mobility declined along with her cognitive abilities.
"Soon," she said, "A bed bath will be necessary."
The very next weekend we fell three times.
Linda came three times a week to spend three hours with her Mom, and Janice came two days a week for three hours. Weekends we were alone for both days.

The first fall occurred on a Saturday morning in the bathroom when she slipped on the tile floor. I had a difficult time getting her up and back to the recliner. Later it happened again, this time in the living room. Every two or three hours I would help her out of the recliner and we would walk through the house. She would look at everything as we walked and close any doors I had left open. It seemed to give her a feeling of being in control when she could close a door or shut a drawer, the things she had always taken care of in the past.

As we strolled through the living room her legs gave out, as if they were made of rubber. She had no control over them and became a dead weight, which I could not hold up. We both went slowly to the floor as her weight took me down with her. The mishap occurred in front of the recliner so putting my arms under hers I lifted and slid her into the chair. On Sunday we fell again while walking through the living room. Again, her legs seemed to turn to rubber and they couldn't hold her up.

After getting her into the rocking chair, I moved the hospital bed away from the wall and pointed it from the corner of the room out toward the center and moved the recliner close beside it so I could more easily move her from the bed to the recliner and back again as needed.

The time had come. The Bath Lady was right.
The moment I had been expecting, and dreading, had arrived. We were looking now at a great lady who would be spending most of the rest of her life in bed.
We knew it was coming but that didn't make it easier.
I moved a recliner close to the bed so I could be close.
How do you get your head around the fact that the end is drawing near for the lady you have been with for sixty wonderful years.

Alzheimer's Disease gets called a lot of things, but the worst of this insidious disease is that it takes you down so slowly and calling it the lingering death, or endless illness probably fits it better than most other names I have heard.

We had decided early on that her hospital bed would be placed in the center of the Living Room so she would always be part of whatever was going on. When visitors came, someone was always sitting by the bed and she was included in discussions, even though she seemed confused by what was happening around her. We moved small shelf units into the room and set them by the walls on either side of the bed. They held all of the supplies needed to care for a bedridden person.

The bed faced the TV so she could watch Murder She Wrote and the Andy Griffith Show for hours on end. When the TV wasn't on the Pandora Music Service provided soft, soothing, Slack Key Guitar lullabies. The music played most of every day. It was good for all of us through these trying times. Several times each day I moved her to the recliner or rocking chair.

The girls decorated the room for each holiday with flowers and

pictures and holiday music would be playing softly in the background

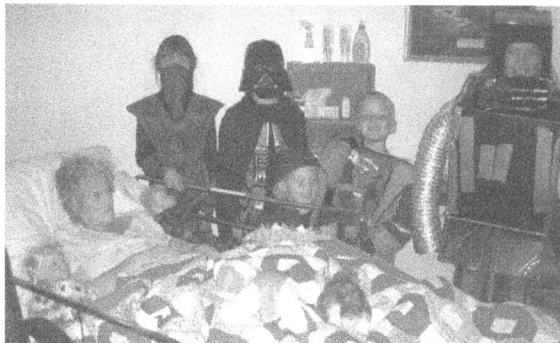

Levi, Julia, Avery, Everett, and Asher show off their Halloween costumes for Great Grandma.

Linda made a small vest with colorful ties that would hold her upright in the rocking chair or wheel chair.
Later the little vests with straps were donated to a 12 year old girl with Muscular Dystrophy.
The family used them to hold her upright in a sled so she could go sledding with the other kids and to help her sit up in her wheel chair the rest of the time.

Lois would have liked it that her vests were put to such good use after she was gone.

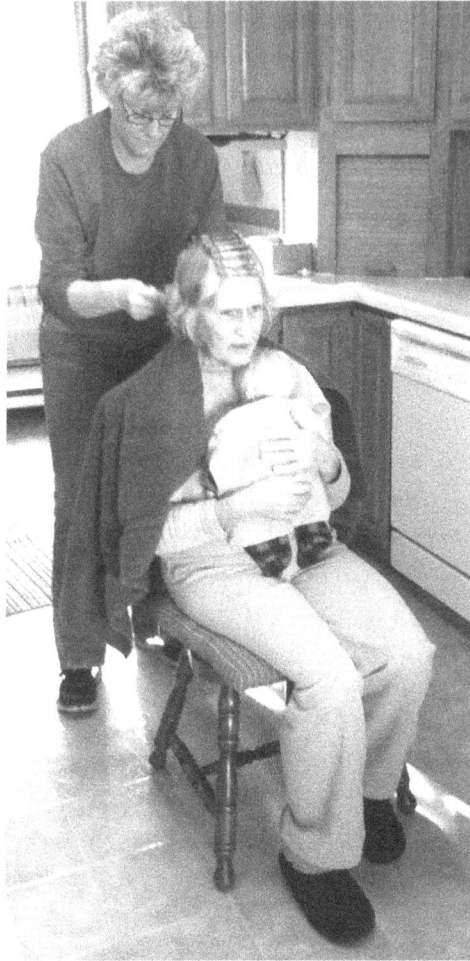

**Lois always wanted to look her best, and the beautician
came to the house to give her a permanent.**

8 - THE ORION LAUNCH

News Flash on TV!

The Orion Launch at the cape has been scheduled. Diana and Ilidio live only forty minutes away from Titusville where I wanted to be the morning of the launch. I packed food and coffee supplies good for a few of days and was off on a new adventure.

The KOA campgrounds at Mims, Florida was the nearest camping site and I arrived early the afternoon before the launch and set up camp.

I plugged an extension cord into the coffee pot before raising the tent to make sure I had hot coffee by the time the tent was up and bedroll unpacked.

The Orion launch was scheduled for 7 AM the next morning and I had been warned to arrive hours early to get a good viewing site.

4 AM came quickly.

Coffee and Ensure was a quick breakfast and the camp breakdown took only a few minutes.

I was off in the pre dawn darkness for Titusville and the Merritt Island Road.

Vehicles were already parking along the highway as I neared the shoreline and I pulled the bike, sidecar and trailer into a parking spot under some power lines. Bad choice but I didn't know it then.

I was parked next to a large RV motorhome. The friendly RV couple invited me to join them in lawn chairs next to the RV which had a large screen TV built into the exterior.

Facing the shoreline I could watch for the live launch, turning toward the RV we could watch the NASA production of the run up to the live launch. These were nice folks.

Others at the viewing site were setting up large cameras on tri pods to record their own memories of this epic event. NASA announced a hold on the launch, then another and another until finally the launch window was closed and the event postponed until the next day.

Disappointed people began pulling out but many of us
stayed to share stories.
We all felt sorry for the couple from New Orleans who had
come for the fourth time to see a launch but each one had
been postponed until it was time for them to return home.
"One more day," John said,, "One more day and we have to
return to our jobs, I hope they go tomorrow."
We heard several similar stories from people who had
driven in from Atlanta, Jacksonville and other cities for
"The Orion" as they began calling it.
As I was showing the sidecar to a guy who came riding in
on a Harley Ultra Glide, I discovered why parking under
the power lines was a bad idea.
Hundreds of gulls used them for a perch and the big spot on
the Harley Dudes leather jacket came as a messy reminder.
I finally called it a day and headed for the Mims KOA
camp for another night in the camper.
Dale Coyner who sold me the camper had sure been right
when he pointed out how easily they could be set up and
how comfortable they were to sleep in.
I made coffee, ate a protein bar and drank a bottle of
Ensure Nutrition drink and was ready for the night.
Same again in the morning.
Coffee, Ensure and protein bar.
A quick but filling breakfast and if it was as good for you
as the ads on TV say I should be as healthy as someone
who started the day with bacon and eggs.
May not have been quite as satisfying, but it was good.
By 4:30 AM I was on the road to Titusville and the much
anticipated launch.
Many of the same people were on hand or just pulling in as
I was and the camaraderie was great.
We watched the latest launch announcements on the RV's
TV and looked through binoculars to get closer views of
the goings on across the water.
When the launch occurred it was, underwhelming.
A brilliant flash of light that moved in seconds into the low
lying cloud cover.

Turning to the TV we could see the Orion flashing skyward, and then, seconds after the flash of light the roar of the rockets reached us.

We watched the flight on TV and listened to the sound as it came to us across the water.

It was a strange experience.

The gathering dispersed quicker this morning as if there was nothing left to talk about.

I took a long, slow peaceful ride through the winding roads of the Merritt Island Wildlife Refuge.

After visiting the wildlife I headed north on A1A the coastal highway for a quick trip up to Flagler's Beach and then moved over to I-95 for the ride back to Lake Mary.

Despite not being able to see the Orion soaring above the clouds, it was a great experience and one more adventure on what some are calling the Long Ride.

The Long Journey, was what one person called the slow trip through Alzheimer's and I couldn't agree more.
I couldn't complain though.

I had family with me nearly every day and all the children, grand children and great grand children shared this long journey with Lois and I.

When Lorna visited Montana with her two children, they along with Hanna and her six children would come and spend an afternoon with Great Grandma.
With eight small great grandchildren playing around her bed, Lois had plenty of company.

She did seem to enjoy watching the kids, even though she could no longer interact with them.

Her eyes would follow them and whenever Hanna lifted the baby up on the side of the bed she did reach out to try and hold him.
When Hanna placed the newest Great Grandchild Zeke next to her on the bed, Zeke placed his hand on hers. It was a touching moment and brought tears to the eyes of some.

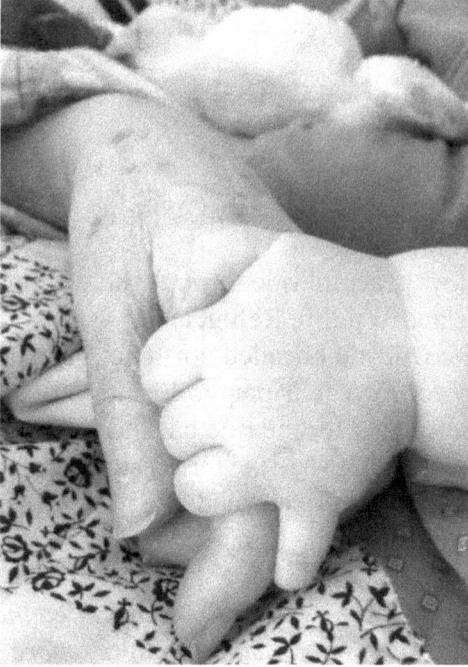

She so loved little kids. They were everything to her all her life, and it showed in the ladies and gentlemen she had raised in our home.

Joni came from Houston several times to spend days or weeks with her Mom.
Being an author meant she could work on her latest book project in the lower level, using the Wi-Fi to stay in contact with editors and publishers.

In the morning she would come upstairs with her ukulele and sing some of the old folk songs they had sung together so many years before.
They both enjoyed the hours spent together.

Although she could no longer sing or react to the music, Lois seemed to relax and have more peace of mind.
Despite the disease, these were good times for all of us.

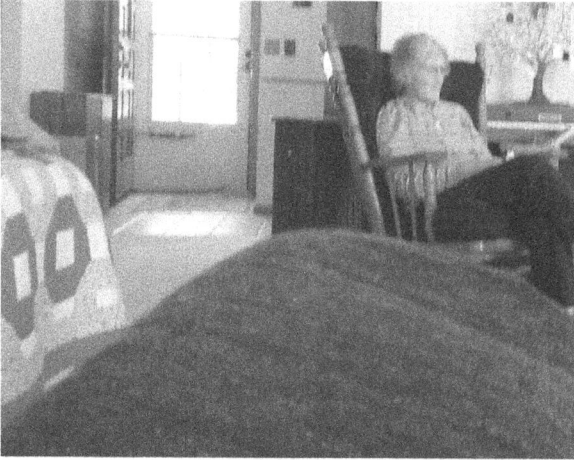

The Bed and Recliner close together

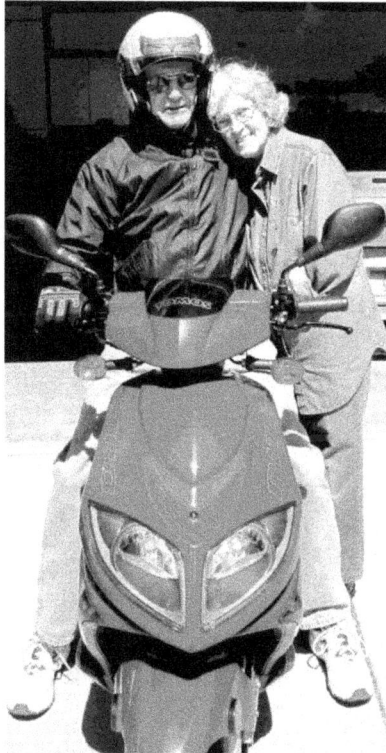

9 - MOTORCYCLE TOUR OF FLORIDA

Autumn days in Florida stayed warm and dry for the most part and I was planning a statewide tour.

The trip began on a bright sunny morning in Lake Mary and took me first to the Kennedy Space Center and then south on A1A to Fort Pierce where I parked at a KOA camp for the night.

Early the next morning I moved on to Highway 70 and traveled westward through the heart of Florida agriculture country. Tree farms, sod farms and orchards.

This was a great ride and at a much slower pace than Interstate travel required.

Through the Okeechobee area with lakes and swamps. Then onto Highway 27 north to Sebring.

Grandson Brian had been pastor of a Lutheran church here and I wanted to get a picture of it to take home.

Lois and I had talked about making a trip to Sebring to visit Brian and his family, but those plans never seemed to come to fruition.

All along the way, as I traveled from Helena, I looked for places that we had talked about visiting "someday." Regrettably, for most of them, the right time, the right day never came, until now.

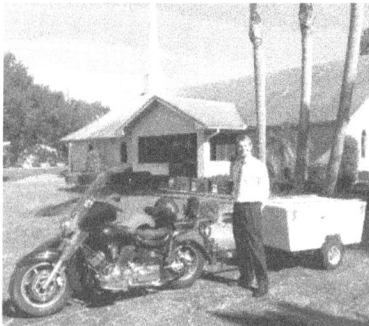

Pastor Luke Willitz, the young Pastor of the New Life Lutheran Church came out to the driveway and asked if he could be of help. He appeared to be slightly puzzled by the appearance of this 80 year old biker who was taking pictures of his church. We had a good visit and then it was back on the road. He is a nice young man.

I stayed that night at the Highland Hammock State park camp grounds.

The previous night at the Fort Pierce KOA had been noisy all night with highway traffic never ending.

Here was a different story.

At this campground, near the city, there wasn't a sound to be heard other than the rustling of the wind in the trees and an occasional owl hooting in the night.

Beautiful area and one I intend to visit again.

I had planned to visit the states west coast and travel over to Naples, Sarasota, St. Petersburg and others.

Alas there were high wind warnings all along the coast and I had no desire to ride my sidecar/tent trailer rig through a high wind area, so I headed north on Highway 27 toward Leesburg, Mt. Dora and Lake Mary.

Not all the trip I had planned, but much of it and I could save the trip down the West coast of Florida for another day, still another adventure.

These were small decisions.

Decisions that didn't require a lot of thought or planning.

So easy when you only have to make decisions that affect yourself and no one else.

One of the hardest decisions we had to make for Lois was when do we need to ask for help from Hospice?

It's the word that so many believe means, this is the end.

The doctor explained that it doesn't necessarily mean this at all, but that a good hospice team can make life easier for the client and the caregivers.

Janice had diligently checked on line and made many phone calls to friends and said she got really good reports on the Frontier Hospice group and suggested we ask the doctor about them.

He was equally impressed with this group, and as we discovered, they would live up to all of the good reviews.

The first visit included a doctor, nurse, social worker and chaplain. They involved Lois as much as possible in questions and explanations.

For people who are apprehensive about calling on hospice for help, I can only say the experience we had was good beyond all expectations.

The Helena, Montana Frontier Hospice was staffed by genuinely caring, loving women and men.

They guided us through each step and stressed that they were always available twenty four hours a day for however long we needed them.

Little did we know at the time that our need would encompass the next 15 months.

The hospice bath lady came every Tuesday and Friday, a nurse came on Thursday, the doctor every four to six weeks, the social worker the same and they repeatedly offered to find a volunteer if I needed time off from the duties of a full time caregiver.

Because I was surrounded by my family support group volunteers were needed only a few times, but they were, like paid staff, caring, helpful people.

Several times I was reminded by the nurses and by Linda that we had to be very watchful to see that Lois didn't develop bed sores or skin tears.

These are common for bedridden people, I was told, and are very painful and difficult to treat.

At one point Linda said, "At the VA hospital we would have the TAP or Turning And Positioning system which makes it much easier to care for the person in bed.

Checking on line I found the system and ordered it. The cost was over $300.00 but it was worth every penny..

It was like a miracle. Using this system I was able to move Lois from bed to recliner and back with a minimum amount of effort required.

The pads for the system cost about $125.00 a month and were well worth it.

Using the TAP system and an air bubble mattress pad we were able to keep her comfortable and avoid the bed sores and discomfort normally associated with spending most of your waking hours in bed.

The TAP system was donated to Frontier Hospice after Lois passed away.

10 - THE HOLIDAYS IN FLORIDA

The Holidays came all too quickly as I continued to make short day trips through North and Central Florida areas. I explored the area along the Atlantic Coast north to Jacksonville and the smaller cities along the way, staying at KOA's or State Parks for a quick overnight trip. Merritt Island with it's miles of narrow winding roads and endless wildlife was a favorite.

Both Thanksgiving and Christmas were marked by the influx of guests to the Sacramento Hotel as some called Diana and Ilidio's home. Each guest brought new stories and questions about "The Ride" and where it would take me when I left Florida.

The build up to Thanksgiving included, what friends called, Diana's famous Cranfest Party. Here each guest was supposed to create and bring to the party, their favorite cranberry dish. There were many, including turkey and other meat cooked with the little red berry as seasoning and many deserts and special drink concoctions.

Most guests, out of kindness I suppose, tasted my offering of a cranberry drink, but there was a lot of it left over when all had left the party. They said it won one of the prizes but I was in the garage showing off my rig to interested guests so I didn't hear the award being made. The Sacramento Cranfest in Florida would rival any taking place in the top cranberry growing areas of Wisconsin and Massachusetts.

Christmas brought more guests and visitors and a visit to the Lake Mary, Florida Christmas Light Park. This park located in the center of the city glittered with every tree, large or small, completely covered with brightly shining lights. This was a great Christmas, and New Years looked like it was going to be great fun.

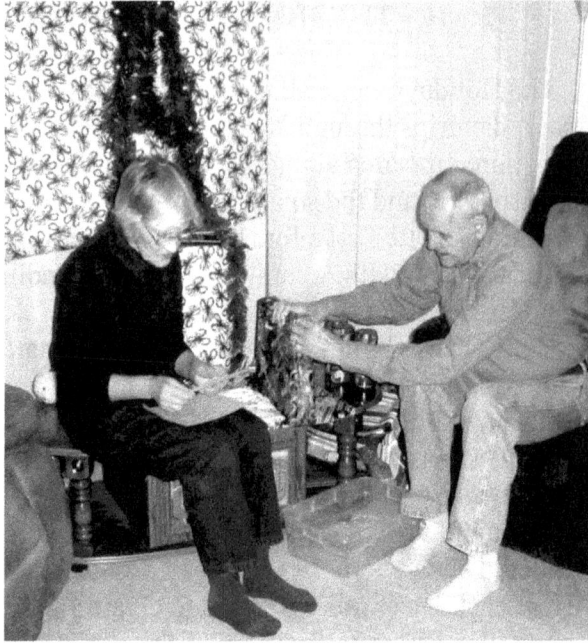

Lois & Del
First Christmas With Alzheimer's

The burning of the Christmas Tree was a custom that Grand daughter Jenny was introducing to the family.

On a chilly New Years Eve I found myself with a small gathering of family and friends on Daytona Beach with a small portable fire pit.

Her boy friend Ben had chopped up several Christmas trees and the fire was started.

Clam Chowder, which Jenny had prepared prior to our trek to the beach, was placed on the fire.

As it cooked we were entertained by the endless New Years Eve fireworks being set off up and down the beach.

The chowder was hot and good and provided warmth against the cool wind blowing in off the ocean. This burning the Christmas Tree could become a great new family tradition.

The trek back to the Sacramento New Years Eve party was quick and many family and friends joined in the fun.

How different from the last New Years Eve.
Roger, Janice and Linda came over to watch the Guy
Lombardo New Years Eve program on TV.
Lois watched with us, but mostly she looked from one to
another and looked at the TV when the music got louder.
Very little reaction to what was going on around her.
I held her hand and she looked at me from time to time, but
I couldn't tell if there was any recognition, of me or the
kids. There were a few tears that New Years Eve.
How different from the days when Lois had the kids tear up
newspapers and put the small pieces in paper grocery bags.
At midnight on New Years Eve, as we watched the ball fall
on the TV, the six kids would shout out the count down and
at midnight would throw their home made confetti in the air
and shout Happy New Year. After a quick clean up of the
newspaper clippings they would be off to bed and Lois and
I would stay up and talk about the old year and the new
year ahead. Different times and different places and far
different from the frail appearing lady who seemed to be so
puzzled by everything going on around her on this New
Years Eve. But on the bright side, she was in her own home
with her own family and was comfortable and seemingly at
peace. Happy New Year?
In many ways yes, despite the downward spiral she was
moving through.

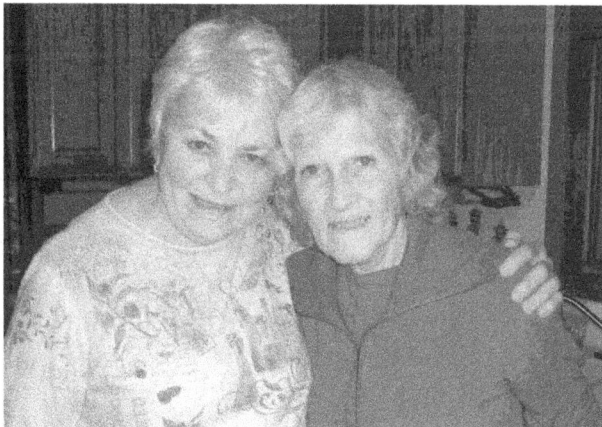

Vivian & Lois

As we moved through each of the many stages of Alzheimer's Disease we were constantly looking for new ways to make her life as easy and comfortable as possible. The music and TV shows both helped, as did family and friends who visited.

Lois' Uncle Harry and his wife Sharon came from Billings several times and my twin brother Dean, his wife Bev and my sister Vivian and her husband Dave all came from Minneapolis. The visits were good therapy, not just for Lois but for the rest of us as well.

When it became apparent that I needed to get a vinyl covered recliner to replace the fabric one Lois had, I mentioned it to the hospice nurse.

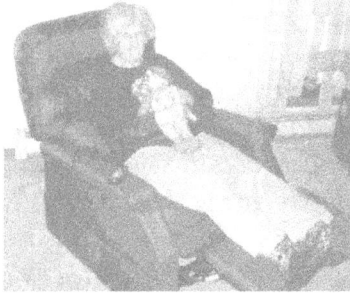

She told me to hold off for a day or to because she had an idea that might help.
A few days later she called to tell me that a national organization called Friends of Hospice would send a check to cover most of the cost. This wonderful group works nationally to assist hospice groups and their clients.
The recliner was all electric and the vinyl covering was easy to clean.
We donated it back to hospice for another elderly person when Lois was gone. Friends of Hospice, is a great organization and offers assistance to many.

It was a new year and Diana had made travel plans.
First on the schedule was a visit to St. Augustine, the oldest continuously occupied city in the USA. It began on a perfect Florida sunshine filled morning.
Temperatures on this third day of the new year were in the 70's and heading in to the 80's.
The drive up Highway A1A through Palm Coast was beautiful with tree lined roads and beautiful houses, condos and retirement communities.

Before we reached St. Augustine we visited a very unique and beautiful National Monument.

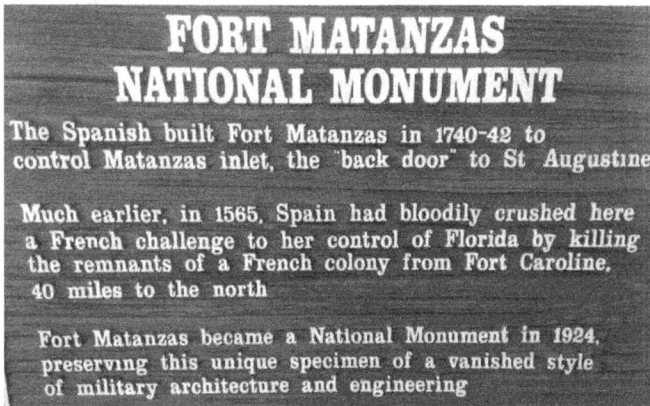

FORT MATANZAS NATIONAL MONUMENT

The Spanish built Fort Matanzas in 1740-42 to control Matanzas inlet, the "back door" to St Augustine

Much earlier, in 1565, Spain had bloodily crushed here a French challenge to her control of Florida by killing the remnants of a French colony from Fort Caroline, 40 miles to the north

Fort Matanzas became a National Monument in 1924, preserving this unique specimen of a vanished style of military architecture and engineering

Fort Matanzas was built by the Spanish in the mid 1700's. The Ranger tour guide explained that the French army had tried to capture the fort, but a hurricane destroyed their ships. Survivors struggled to the shore where they were captured. The Spanish soldiers later executed over 250 French army prisoners.

The fort was originally built to protect the 1500 residents of the village of St. Augustine.

To reach the Fort which is built on an island, Park Rangers use a tour boat to carry visitors across the bay.

Many cannons are on display in the same positions they were placed in when the Spanish fought off French and than English attempts to capture the fort and the city.

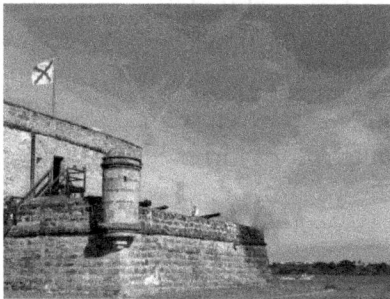

Rangers told visitors to cover their ears as volunteers, dressed in Spanish army uniforms fired one of the cannons. The cannons were capable of hitting ships up to a mile away.

The visit to the Fort Matanzas National Monument
is free and offers visitors a look back in history to the year
1565 when Don Pedro Menendez de Aviles established St.
Augustine as the oldest permanent European city in the
continental United States.
A pleasant beginning for a day filled with blue skies,
sunshine and history.

Following the short boat ride back to the visitors center
we were on our way to the city itself and another National
Monument, Castillo San Marcos. What a place.

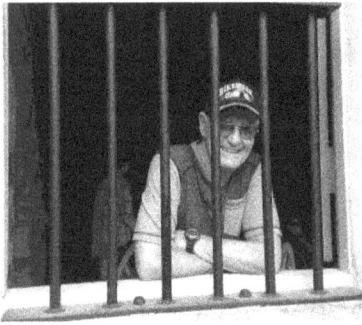

It was built like a castle,
including a moat, and was
used by the 1500 St.
Augustine residents as a
shelter from invading
forces. The fort was also
used as a prison for enemy
soldiers who were captured
in battles with French or
English soldiers.

The bars provided a frame for my picture.

In 1783, following the USA Independence, the English
had to return Florida to the Spanish.
38 years later in 1821 Spain ceded Florida to the United
States. In 1924 Fort Matanzas was named a National
Monument. Care of the facility was transferred from the
War Department to the National Park Service in 1933.

What a great day traveling through some beautiful
scenery and visiting these remarkable US historical sites.
Thanks to Diana's diligent research we had a good time and
discovered a fascinating bit of Florida history.

Lois enjoyed doing research too.
She spent hundreds of hours at the Montana Historical
Society going through micro film newspapers from the
1930's for her book, Fifty Cents An Hour.

*Now she roamed through the house looking for, something.
Always curious and interested in everything around her,
she spent much time at the windows or on the deck which
overlooked the backyard and neighborhood walking path.
Here she could see all kinds of wildlife, as she is doing in
this photo where the deer is peering as intently at her as
she is peering at it.*
The deer were a constant source of enjoyment.
*The deck was a secure place where she was safe and yet
gave her freedom to move outside while we didn't have to
be concerned that she could wander off.*

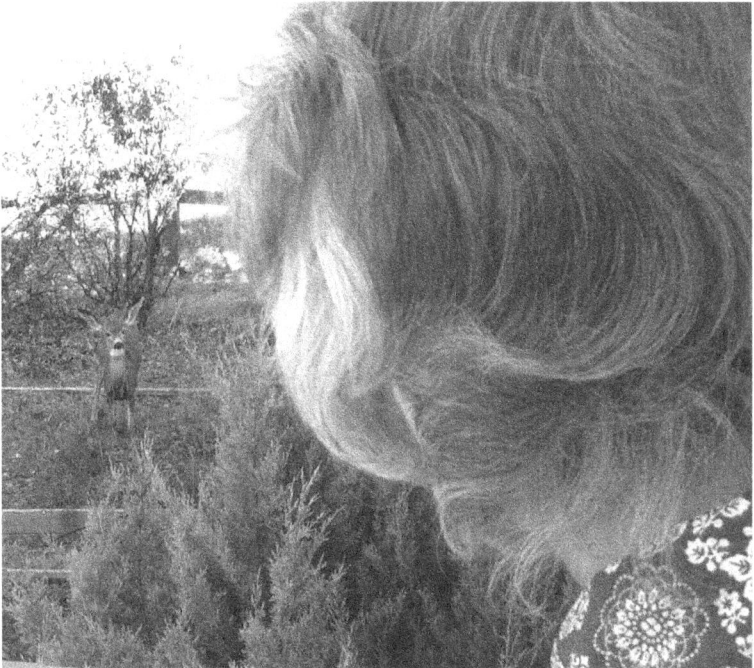

11 - CALIFORNIA HERE I COME

The holidays are over and I'm heading for California with stops in Houston, Roswell, New Mexico and Carlsbad Caverns in the plan.

It was a beautiful sunny day in Lake Mary, Florida and Diana was standing in the driveway waving goodbye as I left behind the comfort of coffee on the lanai every morning, for the long ride to San Jose, California.

I followed the directions VZ NAV was giving me in the Blue Tooth helmet-earphones and found my way out to I-4 and it's connection with I-95 for Jacksonville.
Beautiful day with a few wispy clouds high in the sky and lots of traffic hitting "The 4" northbound.
It was a great day for riding and I was having a great time, in the saddle again for a long road trip.

The ride up I-95 to Jacksonville seemed to take no time at all and I was soon ready to take I-295 west around the south side of the city.
That's when the first big drops of wind driven rain splattered on the windscreen.
What had been a beautiful sunny sky clouded over with swiftly moving clouds.

I stopped under an interstate bridge and pulled on the wet weather gear which would also protect against the wind.
The rain gear always helps but this time, with heavy rain carried by a strong headwind I was still getting wet.
No matter, the temperature was still up so it wasn't a cold rain and the distant horizon showed some blue in it.

The Yamaha was making it's usual comforting rumble as I skirted the edges of Osceola National Forest and then crossed over Twin Rivers and through the spectacular Twin Rivers national forest.
90 minutes later I rode out of the rain and by 3 PM I was pulling into the Tallahassee East KOA at Monticello.

My reservation was good and I was soon checked in and shown to a great camp site.

The Mini Mate tent was up in minutes and several RV'ers strolled over to see this motorcycle-sidecar-tent camper rig being set up. It never failed.

There were curious people wanting to know more about the rig and it's operator and the trip I was on.

Turned into a great way to meet new friends.

My first night back on the road after a two month stay with Diana and Ilidio was good and I slept well, despite the interstate traffic noise.

Coffee, a bottle of Ensure Nutrition drink and a Nature's Valley Protein Fiber Bar got me on the road quickly in the morning and I was on my way to Panama City.

There was a quick stop at a McDonald's for coffee and to use their Wi-Fi to upload pictures and stories to the Face Book group "WITWIG," as some of the Grandkids were starting to call our Face Book Group.

Before the sun reached it's zenith I was turning off I-10 and onto US 75/231 for Panama City.

The beaches looked amazingly the same as when I had moved the family to Florida in 1970.

Despite the hurricanes and rapid growth of the area, there were still sandy beaches and it was fairly quiet as the communities waited for the end of winter and the coming of the thousands of Spring Breakers.

As I rode through Santa Rosa I felt a few sprinkles coming down and pulled into the parking lot of an Ace Hardware store to pull on the wet weather riding gear.

Back on the bike I hit the starter button but to my surprise nothing happened!

I checked for battery lights.

All fine.

Tried the starter button again. Nothing.

My first thought was, the starter clutch.

This model of the Yamaha V Star 1100 was known to have a starter clutch that would give out when least expected.

Entering the hardware store I asked for a phone book and was soon speaking to a tech at Coastal Power Sports in Fort Walton Beach about twenty miles away.

They said they would get me in the shop as soon as I could get my rig to the Fort Walton Beach location.
One call and the AAA Tow truck was on it's way and an hour later we pulled into their parking lot.
The crew took only a few minutes to find the problem.
It was the solenoid and they said they would install a new one and have me back on the road in thirty minutes.

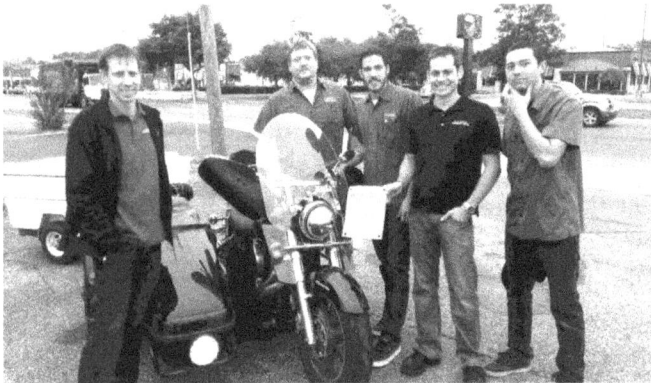

**Crew and Owners of Coastal Power
Sports Fort Walton Beach, FL**

Seeing the "80 year old biker sign" on the back of the rig led to conversation with the crew and the owners of the shop about my long ride and about Lois' illness.
It was a good visit with some easy to visit with bikers.
When they had the bike running once again I went in the shop to settle up the bill, only to hear the owners say:
"No Charge, just get on that rig and ride!"
Here was a team of technicians who knew their job and did it quickly and well.
Business owners who were kind enough to send an old biker back on the road with their "No Charge" statement still ringing in his ears.
Good people and great ambassadors for their community and the biking fraternity.

If you are doing an Iron Butt rider on the road in Florida, and have a bike problem, this would be the right place to call. Coastal Power Sports Fort Walton Beach, Florida

With the machine back in action I rode to the Henderson Beach State Park and set up camp for the night.
Sleep came easily, heart and mind full of thanks for the good people I have met along the way.

Lois would have appreciated this little episode in my journey.
I was making the 16,200 mile trek by myself, but she was not alone on her Alzheimer's journey.
I was with her every day, and children, grand children and great grand children were sharing the journey with us.
How fortunate I was to have such a great support team to share with me each of the many stages this disease took us through.
Health care professionals emphasize in books and articles that caregivers are also at risk and that they should, if at all possible, have periodic breaks from their 24 hours per day care giving duties to preserve their own health.
These breaks were offered me on a daily basis, whether it was Linda, Janice or Roger coming to the house almost daily, Joni coming often from Houston, Diana and Ilidio with their many visits or the weekly phone calls and visits from Allen and Janis. All of these visits in person, by phone or Skype brought assistance in so many ways.
During the moderate stages Lois and Janis would spend hours on the phone. These calls kept Lois in the loop on family matters. As the disease progressed she became less and less aware of things around her and Janis said one of the saddest days of all was the day Mom couldn't talk to her on the phone anymore. Lois' brother Stan said the same thing as they talked every week, until one day she could no longer make the connection.
I handed her the phone and said "It's your brother Stan." She showed no reaction and couldn't talk to him. This insidious disease has lots of hurt for everyone.

12 - Houston - But First A Friendly Wendy's

   Wednesday was to be my long days ride on this leg of the trip. I was on the road early heading for my overnight camp ground stop at Lafayette, LA.
365 miles flew by with only spotty rain showers.
I was glad for warm riding gear to ward off the chill of the cold north wind which had begun midway through the ride.
This was a cold ride through the pan handle of North Florida, Alabama, Mississippi and into Louisiana.
The forecast of a coming Cold Front was right on.

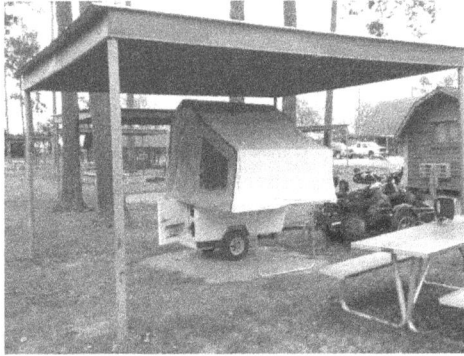

The KOA camp was great and even provided a car port to park the bike and camper under.
By 6 pm the cold north wind brought in the weather front with heavy rain.
This is the coldest night I have spent in the camper and the one night I probably should have opted for a warm, comfortable motel room.
   The morning was gloomy with heavy cloud cover and dense ground fog.
I set out in light rain by 7:30 AM.
Within minutes of getting out on I-10, I was riding in a downpour. This was the heaviest rain I have ridden in yet, and the cold made it even worse.
10 miles down the Interstate I saw an exit and pulled off, hoping to find an awning to hide under.
Better yet, I found a Wendy's Restaurant.
As I pulled into the parking lot I saw a woman coming out the door of the restaurant.
She looked at my rig, shook her head and commented about riding in the cold and rain. When she saw the 80 year old Iron Butt Rider sign she said, "You mean to tell me you rode that thing all the way from Montana?"

She looked at me, looked at the machine and said, "Get in here, I'm buyin' breakfast."
Turns out Shela was the manager and she did indeed buy a biscuit and gravy breakfast for a half frozen old biker.

As I said earlier, I have sure meet some nice people on this long ride across the USA.
Light rain was still falling as I resumed the ride, but it didn't seem as bad now since I was warm and well fed, because of some nice folks at a Wendy's Restaurant.
Thanks Shela, I'll see you on the return trip.
This time I'll buy.

The Google map shows 217 miles from LaFayette, Louisiana to Houston, Texas and I was making good time through the Lake Charles area despite the rain.
The last few miles to the Texas border passed quickly.

As I crossed over into Texas the first ray of sunshine filtered through the cloud cover and minutes later the sky began to clear.
Thanks Texas, I knew you would come through for me.
By the time I arrived at the first Texas Welcome Center, the sun was shining once again and I removed wet weather gear and took a break.

I know my daughter Joni was a little worried about me driving through the city of Houston, so I asked VZ NAV to point me in the right direction to get on the Sam Houston Toll Way and show me the shortest way to the city of Richmond. Here I would find my brother-in-law Stan Smith with whom I would be staying for the next few days.
The GPS did it's job and by using the toll way I avoided most of the city traffic and had no trouble going from I-10 on the Northeast corner of the Metroplex to Richmond on the southwest corner of the city.
Stan had cleared space in the garage for my rig and the trailer, bike and sidecar were soon stowed away and I was settling into a nice room with a good bed.
I felt like saying, "Hooray, I made it through this huge sprawling city with out mishap."
As a matter of fact, I think I did say that.

Coming from Montana which has a population of just under one million people in the entire state, to a city and metro area with over six million people is quite a shock.

After the rainy and cool trip from Orlando to Houston, it was great to see that Texas sunshine and the smiling faces of brother-in-law Stan Smith, with whom I was staying for the week, daughter Joni and her wine making husband Gary, as well as Stan's daughter Shelly, her husband John and son Johnny.

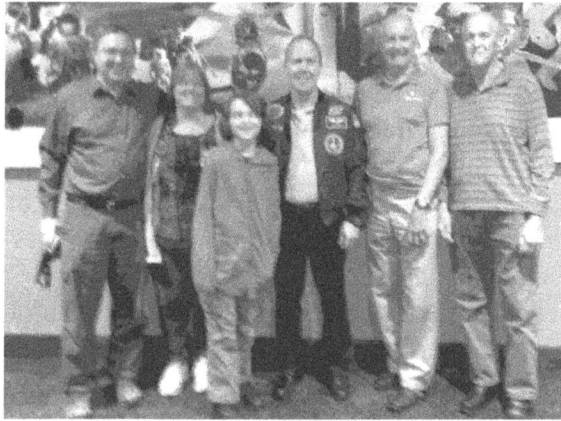

Shelly and John took us to NASA where we toured space exhibits and had lunch with Astronaut Dr. Tom Jones who took time to pose for a picture.
The all day visit included a tour of all the buildings as well as videos and interactive displays.
The NASA visit was great.

The next day Stan and I drove to Austin for a two day visit with his son, Major General Len Smith, the Assistant Adjutant General of the Texas Army National Guard, and his wife Cindy.

The LBJ Presidential Library and State Capitol building were scheduled for visits, but first, the one thing every visitor to Texas should experience:

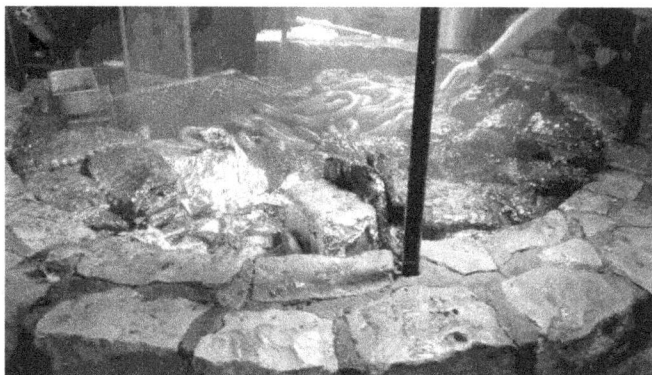

The Salt Lick Barbecue at Driftwood Texas.

Hundreds of people waited up to two hours to be served. The festive atmosphere, music and beer made the waiting an experience in itself.

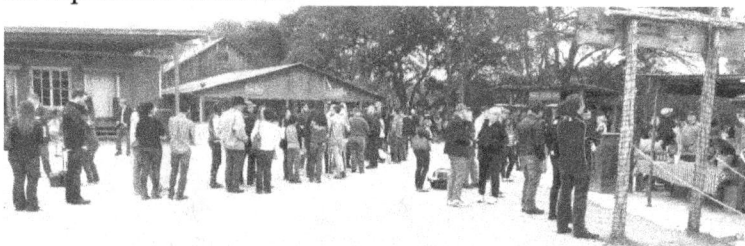

A long awaited adventure was the tour of the LBJ Presidential Library. The building was filled with several floors of picture, videos, sculptures and page after page of his home spun quotations and salty humor.

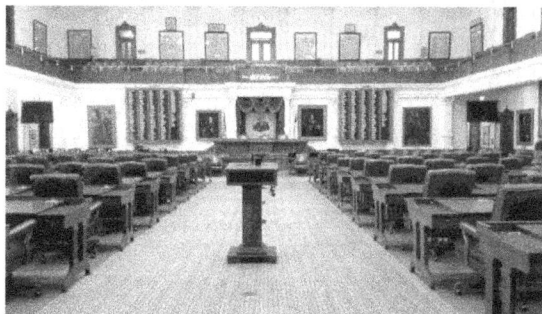

The Legislature was scheduled to begin meeting the next morning at the state capitol and the entire building was buzzing with excitement as each meeting room and office was being readied for the big day. It was a great visit to the Texas Capital City.

73

Back in Houston, Joni had planned still another adventure. She had mentioned to the editors at the Houston Chronicle that her 80 year old Father had arrived in town on his National Motorcycle Tour.

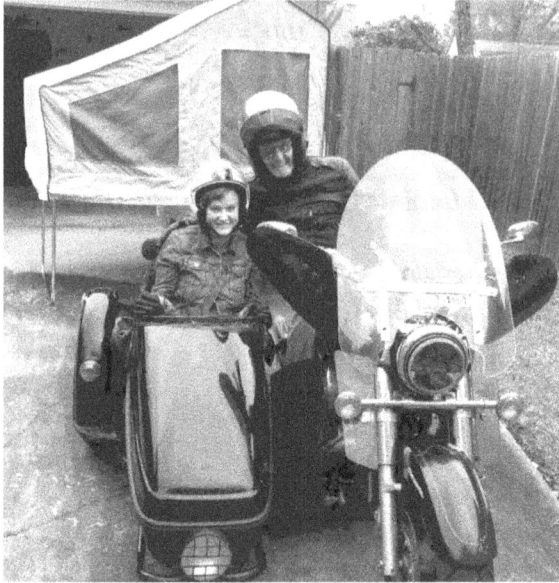

News Reporter Leah & Del

They decided an old guy cruising around the country on a motorcycle with a sidecar and pulling a camper trailer behind it, would make a good feature and sent out a reporter to write the story.

It was a fun interview and I even got to give Leah, the reporter, a ride in the sidecar. Great story on the front page of the Houston Chronicle.

Thanks to Joni for setting that up.

Your contacts in the publishing world amaze me.

13 - Roswell - Carlsbad

Saturday morning I left Stan and a cold Texas rain behind, or so I thought, and headed off toward Kerrville, Texas. After camping in a night that dropped to 31 degrees I renamed it Koolville, Texas.

The south was getting one cold spell after another moving in from the north and I somehow managed to plan my trip so I could camp out in all of them.

That was another night I should have opted for a motel. Fortunately Stan had taken me to a Lowe's Home Center the day before and I purchased a small electric heater. It ran all night and managed to ward off some of the cold.

In West Texas Hill Country and in New Mexico, towns are not too close together, so before crossing the state line into New Mexico, as I was running very low on gas I needed to find a service station.

There didn't seem to be any towns near enough on the Interstate so I took a chance, pulled off I-10 and headed for the small town of Harper, Texas 18 miles away.

I made it, but I was running on fumes before I got there Everything worked out well though as it was Sunday morning and a small white church had a service that was about to begin.

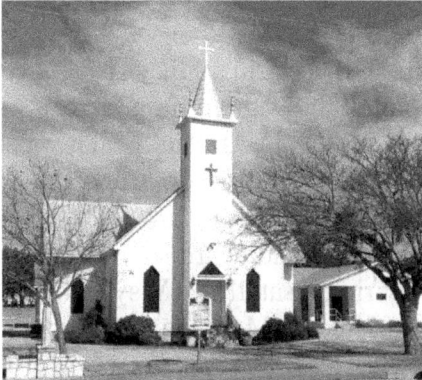

I walked in during the first hymn and was made to feel right at home despite the black leather jacket and biker clothes. They had no organist but did have two good guitar players, one of whom had a great voice.

He led the song service with great easy to sing hymns. What a beautiful service at St. James Lutheran Church in the small town of Harper, Texas.

This was turning out to be a great day and a beautiful ride.

Then it was off on I-10 to Fort Stockton, on my way north to Roswell, New Mexico.

First though I made a quick stop in Pecos, Texas.
As I passed through Pecos I stopped long enough to get a picture of the sign for the worlds first rodeo.
How cool is that?

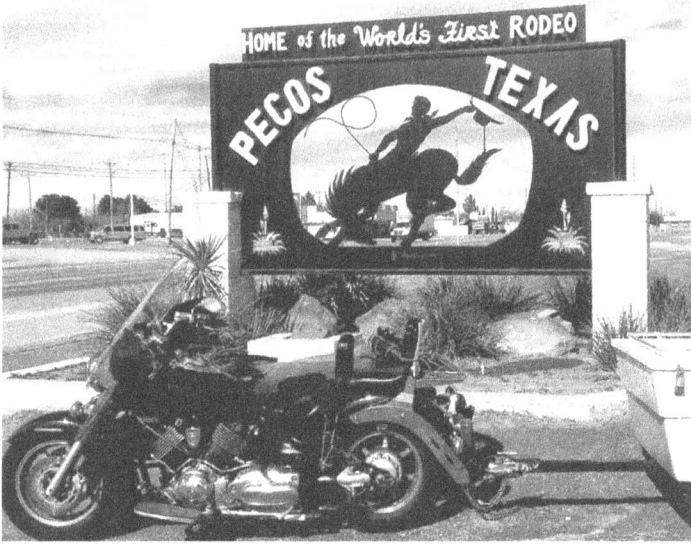

Pecos, Texas, home of the world's FIRST rodeo. How about that. Glad I spotted that sign in time to get a picture. Camping was great at a KOA in Artesia, which was half way between Roswell and my next stop, Carlsbad.

By morning I was ready to visit the famed UFO Museum and research Center which I had heard so much about.

Years ago while rewiring a satellite TV system at a house in the North Valley of Helena, Montana, the home owner introduced himself.

Dr. Jessie Marcel was a man I had read about years earlier. He was 12 years old in 1947 when his Father, a Major in the US Air Force was the first member of the military to view the site where a reported UFO had crashed.

His Father brought pieces of the craft home to show his son at 2 AM in the morning.

Hours later, other Air Force officers picked up the alleged UFO fragments and took them away. Although first reports from the base information office referred to it as a UFO, the air force soon put out a news report that it was a weather balloon. Dr. Marcel said, "some people don't believe I saw pieces of a UFO, but I know what I saw and it was not of this world." He never wavered from that belief.
One of the exhibits showed the early news paper stories.

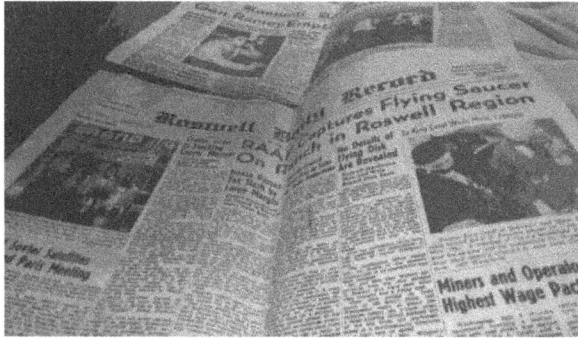

I spent several interesting hours at the UFO Museum. It is well done with tasteful, thoughtful exhibits and presents a clear picture of both Government and Private UFO Research. The $3.00 admission seemed very reasonable and I said so to the lady at the desk. She said it is to make the facility available to all. Great concept.

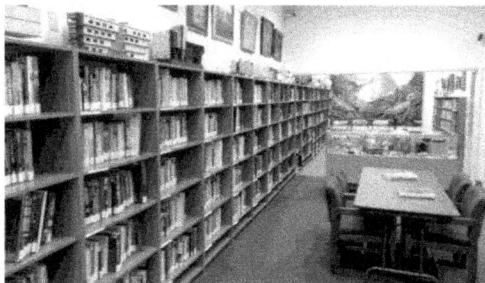

The UFO Museum Research Center

Following a great visit at Roswell, NM and tour of the UFO Museum I headed for Carlsbad Caverns.
My Golden Passport Senior Citizen Pass worked again.

The Caverns are deep and cool.
I purchased a sweat shirt to wear on the tour.
The tour itself lasted an hour and a half and provided an in depth look at the fantastic rooms and all of the giant columns of stone which had been carved in to beautiful sculptures.
It is beautiful, but pictures I took just don't do it justice.

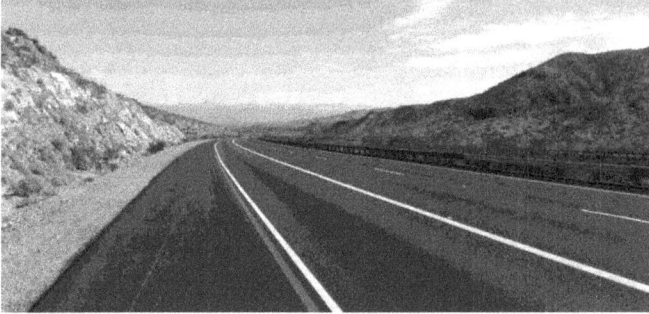

The surrounding countryside is also spectacular with boulders jutting out from every hillside and making the miles long drive into the caverns, a great drive.
The narrow, winding entry road is a great motorcycle ride.
I filled up at the only gas station near the caverns and turned onto the southbound highway, US 62.
The sign said 166 miles to El Paso.
   I knew this was going to be tight on gas, even with the reserve gas can I have on the back of the sidecar.
The road to El Paso was long, with many hills, but not a lot of curves. A good ride.
   Dry and sunny, this was a good change from the days of rain I had on my way to Houston and while I was in Houston.
Seemed like the rain was following me across the south.
   As the city of El Paso drew closer, it seemed I might make it without going to the spare gas can.
Didn't happen.
   Some 20 miles out of the city I sputtered to a stop.
It's nice to have the spare can of gas, but even nicer if you never have to use it.

This time I had used up the reserve and reached for the spare. Glad to have it too.

Sure beats having to walk to a service station that appears to be miles away.

The day before I had stopped when I saw a biker sitting under an overpass with his Harley Davidson Sportster.

Out of gas, he said, "I have been sitting here for five hours and no one would stop."

I filled his tank with two gallons of Chevron Premium and when he insisted on paying me I told him no, just pass it on to the next guy.

He was one happy biker when I left.

The next day as I was nearing Tucson, the rains came again. Light at first, but hard enough so that I pulled off at Benson, Arizona, some 45 miles east of Tucson.

Bypassing the camp grounds and a rainy night in the Mini Mate camper I checked into the Days Inn motel.

The heavy rain was supposed to last for two days so I booked the room for two nights.

By mid-afternoon of the second day the forecasters had added another day of heavy rain to the forecast so I elected to stay for a third night.

TV News was full of stories of "Swift Water Rescues," and reports of 8 inches of rain in the nearby mountains.

Washes, gullies and creeks were overflowing.

Many people were being rescued from flooded cars.

The motel room was a good place to be during what the motel clerk called, "a good old fashioned gully washer."

It certainly was that.

In the early days of our long life together Lois always loved the rain.

Growing up as she did in North Eastern Montana where rain was often sparse, she enjoyed the rain and talked about how everything would come to life after the storm.

As the Alzheimer's Disease progressed through each stage, her fear of thunder, lightening and rain storms caused new reactions and more reminders about the course her health was taking.

One Alzheimer's web page lists three stages of the disease. They say that Alzheimer's Disease progresses slowly through three general stages.

A pamphlet from Alzheimer's Association, ALZ.org lists seven stages and has the most complete descriptions of each stage that we have seen. It is handed out free from many medical offices and health care groups.

Researching I found several web sites that said there are seven stages and one that indicated they thought there were 31 stages to watch for.

They all had suggestions and offered to help with pamphlets, magazine articles and studies, but practical How-To-Do-Home Care assistance was hard to find. Primarily because as they point out, every one is different and each person reacts to the disease in their own way.

Because Lois had always been such a great "hands on" Mother, all six of the children are capable of looking at a problem and figuring out a solution.

This is what happened when they were confronted with the totally unexpected illness of their Mom, and the strange effect it was having on her day to day living.

They, each in their own way, looked for things they could do to keep her comfortable and to help me with the care giving job.

We all came to the conclusion that when you do the caregiving out of love, it is much easier.

All who entered Lois' space, felt that love.

14 - Tucson to San Jose

The sun was bright by Sunday morning. The storm was over and I was ready to ride.

But wait!

I was headed for Phoenix, and it was Super Bowl Sunday. I searched the internet for highways that would give me the widest distance from the Super Bowl Mania and found it on I-8, some 40 miles south of Phoenix. Turning onto The 8, I headed west away from the big game.

Great ride and many signs directed me to the best Phoenix by-pass highways.

To my surprise, traffic was light as I bypassed Phoenix, traveled to Yuma on I-8 and took Highway 85 north to get back on I-10.

Apparently everyone who was heading for the Super Bowl was already there.

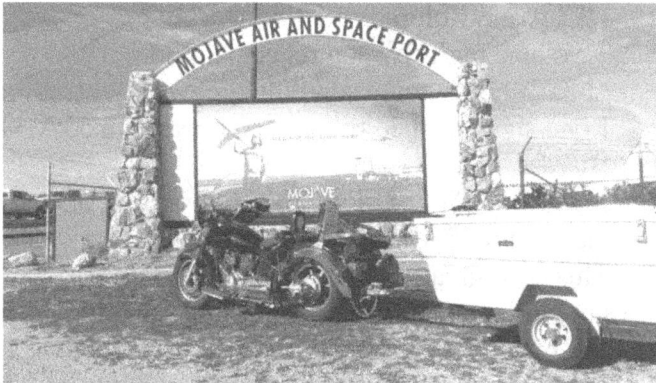

Mojave Arizona Spaceport!

That's what the sign said, and of course I had to pull off and see what was going on out here in the middle of the desert.

There were space flight schools, training services of all kinds and even a "Boneyard."

A place where they park out of service airplanes of all kinds for storage.

I was aiming for Blythe, California where I would get off I-10 and drive north toward Needles, California on US 95 but by the time I reached the Arizona border I was tired enough to look for a camping site.
I found it at Quartzite, Arizona.
The Desert RV Campgrounds was a big difference from the state campgrounds and the KOA's I have been frequenting along the way.
 The office was closed on weekends and registration was by placing a ten dollar bill in the envelope and sliding it through a slot in the door.
  The tent camp area was an open area of sand and gravel. This is what they mean by "Dry Camp."
No water or electricity, just a place to camp for the night.
And not a bad night at that.
Quiet and warm,
 The next days ride from Blythe, California to Needles carried me through some great scenery along the Mojave Desert and Colorado River.
Two lane highway at a relaxed speed.
  I have just learned something new about California.
Road signs warned trucks of a maximum 55 MPH.
BUT!
Signs also warned any vehicle towing a trailer of a maximum 55 MPH speed limit.
This is so great.
I'm pulling a Mini Mate tent camper behind the motorcycle.
 I HAVE to drive slowly through this beautiful area.
When the speed limit is 75 and I'm driving 65 I feel guilty for impeding traffic.
But here, the State of California is ORDERING me to drive at a nice relaxing 55 MPH.
It is great and this law for towing vehicles extends across the entire state.
Worked well as I drove through the coastal mountain range approaching Santa Margarita.

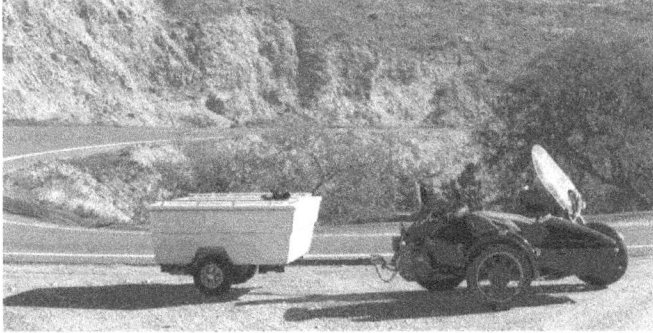

Suddenly, Highway 58, a narrow two lane road began climbing via switch backs signed at 10 to 15 MPH. Sharp turns appeared as I looked down at drop offs several hundred feet down.
No Guard Rails!
As I slowly wound my way up the mountainside the drop offs were deeper and deeper and the turns seemingly sharper and slower.
It was a GREAT ride.
But still a relief to reach the top and make my way down the back side and into a beautiful little town called Santa Margarita. The KOA camp was 8 miles out. I camped by the shores of Santa Margarita Lake.
It was so quiet I could hear the frogs along the lake shore.
What a beautiful night of camping.
From Santa Margarita, I turned north on Highway 101 and rode slowly through the agricultural heart of the state.
It was a fantastic ride to San Jose.
Mile after mile of orchards and fields of vegetables.
The countryside was alive.
Farm workers in the fields and irrigation water flowing. This is the real California. Beautiful.

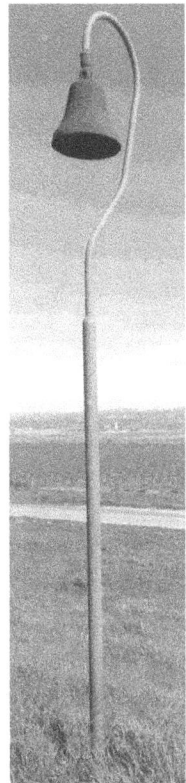

It was here that I saw the first of the mile marker bells along the highway.

The Mission Bell Mile Markers started in 1906 along the El Camino Real. The state legislature assigned the task of keeping the bell project alive to the Department of Transportation.

The bells are a unique and historic feature of Highway 101. What a great idea to keep history in front of travelers through these beautiful bells.

Finding the Klebig home in San Jose was easy with the VZ NAV working fine.

The odometer turned over 19,000 miles as I pulled into the Klebig driveway.

About 11,000 miles from where I started this epic ride last Sept. 27th.

Great adventures continue as I leave in two weeks for the return trip to Orlando and Lake Mary, Florida.

Then, when the warm air returns to the mountains of Montana I will complete the ride I started almost six months earlier.

Home is starting to sound pretty darn good after all of these miles on the road and the many nights in the tent camper.

15 - California - What A Great Experience

It was a grand welcome from the Klebig family and they had many plans for the next couple of weeks. High on my "to do" list was a visit to the world famous Computer History Museum, which Janis had written many of the diorama scripts for.

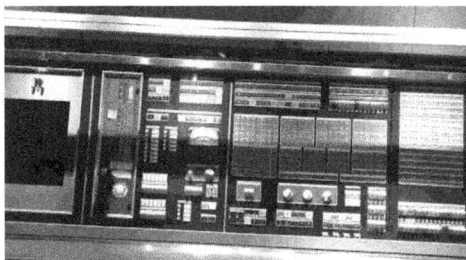

The museum has hundreds of exhibits detailing the history of computers going back hundreds of years.

The work of World War Two decoders trying to break the enemy codes and through their efforts, shorten the war. There were demonstrations of working computers that could fill a room with the wiring and amplifiers that it took to make them operate.

Ever present in modern computer history is Google and

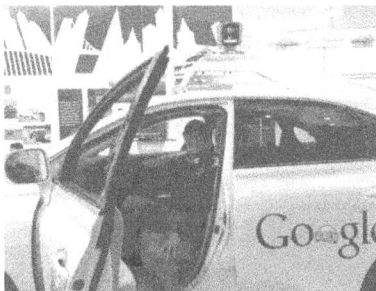

here was the car that could drive itself. The car is open and anyone who wants to get in and see what it looks like from the inside may do so. Grandson Vaughn said he had seen it in action driving down a San Jose street. The museum visit took hours and we were still unable to see it all. This is one California destination point anyone who is trying to make sense out of this new computer age should see.

The museum building is worth the visit by itself.

Lois would have enjoyed the visit to the computer museum as she enjoyed writing and researching her books and other writing projects.

It was hard to see the skills she had used on all of these projects slowly fading away.

Through the moderate stage of the disease she kept using her computer and working at her projects.

It must have been very hard for her to be unable to continue work on her new book.

The research had been done and now the task of writing the book was to begin.

The computer files confused her.

I had set up an icon on the desktop of her computer and she would click on that and bring up the files she needed.

Weeks after she passed away I was looking through boxes of her first book, Fifty Cents An Hour - The Builders and Boomtowns of the Fort Peck Dam.

I discovered over 500 copies of the book had been signed. It was an amazing discovery.

When she brought up the files for her new book, she became confused and couldn't remember what she needed to do next. At that point she would apparently, turn to her work table and begin doing the one thing she could remember how to do.

She signed copies of Fifty Cents an Hour.

She had inserted in the front of the book a picture of a tree and called it "her signing tree."

She opened the books to the page with the tree and carefully signed each one. She then placed the signed copies back in the boxes.

550 books had been signed, it was one thing she could still remember how to do.

To be busy doing something was always important to her and even with the fading skills and memories it brought peace and perhaps even a bit of happiness to know that she could still do this one thing that needed to be done.

We came down off the snow covered mountain at Lake Tahoe, Jordan, Vaughn and me. They had a great day on the slopes and I a great day writing and people watching.

People of all ages, including many senior citizens were having a beautiful sunny time riding the gondolas and taking advantage of a warm winter day.

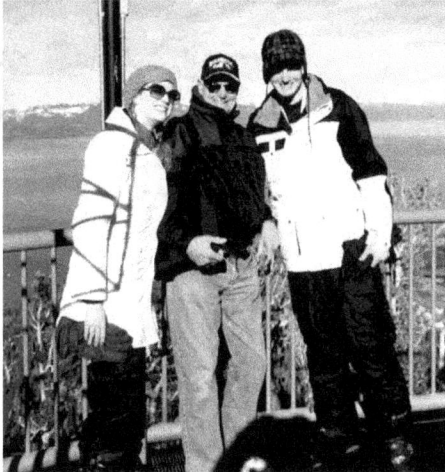

Riding the lifts to ever higher levels was a thrill and took us to a point high on the mountainside where the view went on forever

Dinner was a special buffet where you filled your bowl with the your choice of a wide variety of items, gave it to one of the chefs working around the Mongolian Stir Fry cooking center and watched as they twirled their spatulas in ever more complex patterns and then with a flourish scooped everything on to a platter and told you to enjoy. The two young men were great and I was surprised when Vaughn said they were trainees who worked the quieter week nights until they were skilled enough to handle the weekend crush of visitors.

A meal to remember - a day to remember.

Thanks to Grandson Vaughn and Granddaughter Jordan for a fantastic day on the hill.

It's Here!

The certificate showing I had successfully completed the Saddlesore 1000-1 and was now a certified member of the Iron Butt Association had arrived at the Klebig residence.
 It had been mailed to my home mailbox in Helena, Montana and Linda had sent it on to San Jose.

I was now a certified member of this great organization.

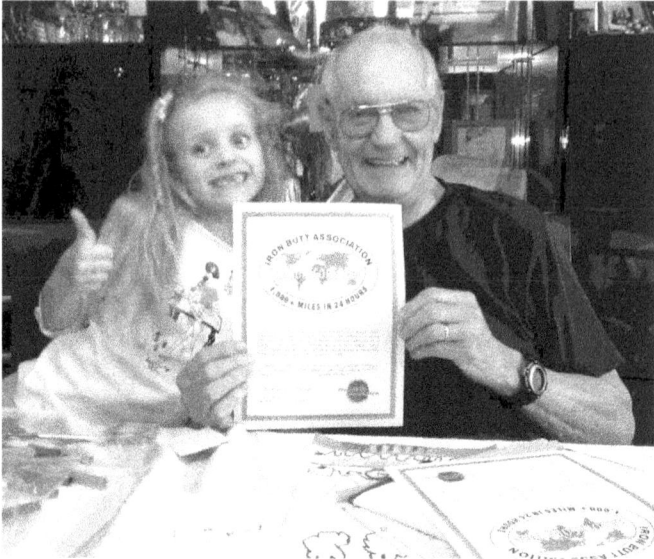

Del with Great Grand daughter Miley

Sunday is a special day for the Klebig family at Apostle's Lutheran Church.
Vaughn heads up the Praise Music Team and after a week night practice session, they lead the music on Sunday.
Vaughn playing rhythm guitar and bass, Jordan on piano and Mike on guitar lead a team of great musicians and the music is fantastic.
What a beautiful Sunday morning.
As I continue my ride through the south, the songs they sang play back in memory for many days.
After church, lunch is at a downtown San Jose Food Mall and included a meeting with Pratima and Atul, the Mother and Brother of Vaughn's girl friend Pooja. Great folks and we had a nice visit.
A special treat was a ride in the Road Trek van down the coast on Highway 1.

Janis thought I should see what Highway 1 was like and wanted me to see Big Sur and other points along this road which is a legend among bikers everywhere.

It lived up to everything I had heard and read about it and by days end I was even more anxious to get back on the bike and "ride the twisties" as bikers like to call it.
My California visit is all too soon drawing to a close.
I plan on reversing my course and going back to Florida, and then, weather permitting I will set out for the final leg of my 16,000 mile ride, back to Montana.

During my San Jose visit I prevailed upon Mike to go with me to the Verizon store to choose a new IPhone to replace my nearly worn out Windows Smart phone.
The IPhone 6 was the choice and he walked me through it's operation to the point I felt I could use several of it's primary features and apps.
Thanks to Mike for making my homeward trip easier through his knowledge of electronics.
Monday morning found me taking the first leg of my trip back home to Montana.

From San Jose, SIRI, the lady who runs my new IPhone 6, took me to Castroville and on to the bikers favorite road, the fabled California Highway 1.

What a ride it was down the Pacific Coast to San Luis Obispo, or SLO, as the locals refer to it. The road winds in and out of shoreline views and you ride through an ever changing up and down countryside, all the while watching a shoreline of sandy beaches and rocky inlets.
Cars were parked at every "Vista Viewing Area," and the already narrow highway became even narrower.
Many bikers were riding the twisties.

The KOA camp at Santa Margarita was a great rest stop overnight as I prepared for a ride through the coastal mountain range on Highway 58. This was the same mountain highway I had ridden on my way to San Jose and I wanted to ride through it with bright morning sunshine lighting up the hills and valleys.

I was looking forward to my ride through some of the windingest, twistingest mountain roads I have ever ridden.
  ALAS!
My morning ride through the twisties began in a dense, heavy fog that was almost like rain.
The coastal fog I had been warned about completely enveloped the mountainside.
The winding mountain ride was a thrill and the sun burned off the fog when I was about half way through the hills.
  I rode US 58 to Bakersfield where I took a short ride on Buck Owens Boulevard and a few blocks on the street called Meryl Haggard Way.
Country music lovers know those two names and I took time for a short ride down the streets named after these country music superstars.

  Picking up I-40 I was soon on my way to Barstow.
It was a good ride all the way to Barstow where the KOA was easy to find and was nice and quiet.
Morning came with bright California sunshine.
  Life is good.

16 - Route 66

My son Roger had urged me to ride at least some of the fabled highway called:
ROUTE 66 !
The National Historic Trails designation made it sound like a well loved highway.

And perhaps it is in some areas, but San Bernardino County and the city of Barstow seem to have forgotten it's value as a tourist attraction.

It started out well with ten miles of good road but then the asphalt became so broken up it was an impossible ride. Like other riders before me, I took to the sandy shoulder and rode the next eight miles at 15 to 20 miles an hour, dodging the ruts carved into the sandy shoulder by previous History Buff riders.

The sign saying, "I-40 East" looked very welcome and I made the switch from the rutted, broken up asphalt to the interstate and was soon running at 55 MPH on a good road. 35 miles from Barstow I pulled off the interstate to visit "The Route 66 Oasis," for gas.
$5.25 per gallon Premium!
Whoa, it wasn't that pricey back in the days when they were shooting the TV series.

At this point I moved back onto Route 66 and had a good ride on this section of the old road.
Here the fabled highway wound it's way through 140 miles of desert, including the Hualapai Indian Reservation, heading for Kingman, Arizona.
The road was good and I had a lot of time to think about the old TV series and the history behind this well traveled highway. Burma Shave Signs brought back memories.
After the Route 66 experience the ride to Kingman went quickly as I was back on I-40.
The KOA was big and well equipped with fenced in tent camper sites which included water and electricity.

The latter was needed for the electric heater since the temperature had dropped to 27 degrees by morning.

The planned visit to the South Rim of the Grand Canyon was put off as another cold spell moved in from the North.
I made a bee line for the Phoenix suburb of Surprise, AZ where I found a big welcome and a warm room waiting at the home of my Cousin Lynn Weaver.
The rear brakes on the motorcycle seemed to be fading as I rode into town.
Fading brakes are not something you want to see when you are riding through the western mountains.
Especially when those brakes are stopping, not only the motorcycle, but also a sidecar and a 300 pound Mini Mate Tent camper.
Lynn knew of a nearby Yamaha dealer where a first rate service department took the machine in, even though it was after 3pm on a Friday afternoon.
The brake pads were good so the crew flushed the brake lines and cylinder and I am stopping better than ever.
Fortunately for me, Lynn is a biker and knew where to take the machine and we were able to get it taken care of in a timely fashion.
Saturday morning Anna was up early preparing a great breakfast of sausage, eggs and toast. What great folks to take in an itinerant biker and make him feel right at home.
Mid day Saturday I headed for Phoenix and rode I-10 around the city in the busy Saturday morning traffic.
Four lanes of fast moving traffic doesn't seem to bother me as much as it did a few months ago.
From Jason leading me through the Monday morning Washington DC traffic, to Diana & Ilidio leading me through Miami, Joni and Stan advising on Houston traffic, and the Klebigs showing me what real traffic is in San Jose, I have a lot more confidence.
All the same, it was a relief to find the road to Tucson a whole lot quieter and with less traffic except through the City of Tucson itself.
Scenery is fantastic. I think I have seen about every kind of mountain range the country has to offer.
Pulling off the interstate I camped at Benson Arizona, 45 miles east of Tucson.

I decided to stay an extra day since a cold spell that would make camping less than comfortable was moving into New Mexico and Texas during the night.

I booked the second night at the same Days Inn that had kept me dry during the rainstorm I encountered on my way out to California.

Meanwhile I discovered a nice little Lutheran church near Benson. It was in a valley on the west side of town, a couple of miles out, and the name seemed appropriate.

Peace In The Valley Lutheran.

Nice folks.

The 2006 Yamaha V Star 1100cc Classic had 8,300 miles when I bought it in August 2014.

It turned over 20,550 as I left the church parking lot.

What a grand adventure this visit to our widely spread out family has been.

And what great people I have had a chance to visit.

The two minute set up of the tent camper took two hours last night as a steady stream of RVers stopped by to hear all about it.

One woman went rushing over to get her Mom, Dad and two brothers so they could see it too. They took pictures and web addresses where they could find more information. I told them to look for Dale Coyner who did such a great job getting me set up for camping.

A hard to understand gentleman from Montreal spoke both French and English while discussing camping in his RV.

He saw the 80 year old rider sign on my bike and said, "Well, how old do you think I am?"

I told him he didn't look a day older than 70 years.

He said, "Well I hope not, I'm only 61!"

Hmmm, I actually thought he looked older than me.

Must have been his beard and mustache.

He left then, I guess he didn't want to talk camping any longer and he was moving a lot faster when he left then when he came. Strange.

Tucson/Benson, Arizona behind me now and I'm heading for Las Cruces, New Mexico.

Windy ride.

Winds running 25 to 35 MPH and gusting even higher, I'm really getting bounced around.

Big rigs sailing by me bring more wind gusting.

What a ride.

I pulled off the road early at Deming, NM and called it a day.

Didn't even try to set up the tent camper, and pulled in to a Days Inn instead.

The motel room was big and most important, out of the wind.

Should be a better ride tomorrow.

  And indeed it was.

The wind had turned and I was riding in the cradle.

A great tail wind behind me and the machine was running swift and easy.

I made a quick stop at the Lordsburg, New Mexico McDonald's for coffee and to use the great McD's WiFi. I keep trying to update the kids Facebook Group,

"WITWIG" as often as possible and McD's is the quickest place to do that.

Not this time though.

The big guy with a full set of leathers looked over from another table and said, "Mind if I join you?"

He brought his coffee over and asked about my ride.

"I parked next to your rig, and that is quite a set up."

I told him where I had been and where I was going and asked about his ride.

 "DR 650," he said.

Now I knew there would be a story here.

The DR 650 Suzuki is not only a great street bike, it handles the off road runs too.

"I'm on my way home to British Columbia after riding all the way to the southern tip of Argentina."

 WOW! and I thought I was doing a long ride.

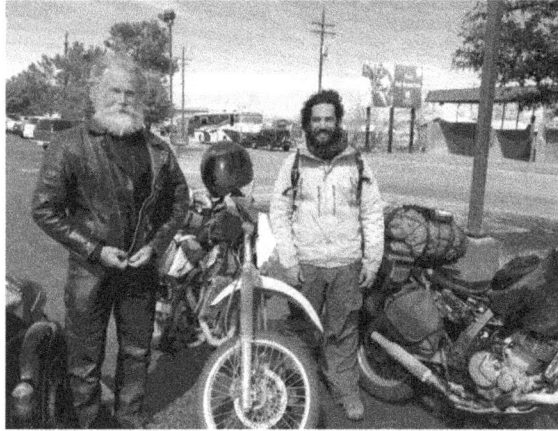

At that point a young rider sitting at another table came over and asked, "Did you say DR 650? That's what I'm riding too."

Double WOW! I could see another story coming on.
I said "Where has your ride taken you?"

He said, "I made it as far as Costa Rica, but money started running low so I'm on my way home to BC too."

Here were two kindred spirits, running their own ride, doing there own thing, but meeting at a McDonald's Restaurant in the middle of New Mexico.

Bob Weeks was a tall guy with gray hair and beard. Tom Trautmansdorf was a young guy with black hair and beard. They had fulfilled whatever dream it was that took them from Canada through the USA and into South America. What fantastic stories they would have for their children and grand children.

As we talked other customers seemed to gravitate into the section we were sitting at and seemed to move even closer to hear the biker stories that were being shared by three strangers in the middle of New Mexico.

I finally had to say, "Guys I have really enjoyed meeting you and hearing your stories, but I have to move on, the family in Houston is expecting me."

And so I left, but I knew I would never forget my chance meeting with Bob Weeks and Tom Trautmansdorf.

Great guys and they had both made gutsy rides, through some rough country.

Rides that most of us would never dare to make.

I knew I would be stopping off in Kerrville and Fort Stockton before seeing the smiling faces of Joni, Gary, Stan Smith and the others in Houston so I needed to get back on the road.

 West Texas Hill Country, they call it.

 It's a long way between towns in West Texas.

Lots of miles, rolling tree covered hills to see and interesting people to visit with.

This was a long ride day.

 360 miles across New Mexico and into Texas with a tail wind lending strength and speed to my machine.

Rode into Kerrville at 4:30 but another chance meeting with a couple of interesting bikers held me up.

Howard Wong and Brian Rudy were Vancouver British Columbia attorneys who had planned ahead for a great ride through the southern USA.

A few months earlier when all was warm and sunny, they had ridden their Harley Davidson machines to San Luis Obispo in southern California and put them in storage.

Now as the cold of winter held sway over their homeland, they took a plane ride to California, got their bikes out of storage and began a ride which would take them to San Antonio, Austin and other Texas cities and might even lead them to Daytona for the Bike Week gathering in March.

Howard Wong and Brian Rudy

What were the odds that I would meet four people from British Columbia in the wilds of New Mexico and Texas, and that they would each have their own dream and their own ideas about what constituted a great ride through this fantastic land we call America.
Great people. Great rides.

Fort Stockton was a Texas city I had stayed in when I was heading west.
Now, on the eastern run, I decided to go right on by and try to make it to Hammond, Louisiana.
Yesterdays tail winds had changed in to South East head winds with occasional heavy rain squalls.
Arriving in Hammond, I pulled in to the parking lot of a Days Inn and was happy to hear they had a room left for a cold and wet biker.
I was soaked through. Even my waterproof boots were soaked and I could wring water out of my socks as I held cold feet in front of the electric heater I carried in the rig.

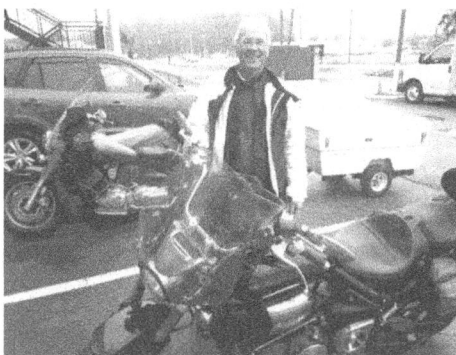

Stepping out of the motel room door I met another biker headed for Daytona Beach and Bike Week.
Guido was from Switzerland and had borrowed a US friends Yamaha for a ride through the south.
Wearing his Frog Togs wet suit he had managed to avoid some of the weather but not all.
He was also in the process of drying out wet clothes.
He had a secret for keeping his feet dry.
Without waterproof boots he knew he would have wet feet so he slipped each foot into a plastic grocery bag and then slipped the plastic covered feet into his riding boots.
The boots got wet but his feet stayed dry.

Great idea Guido and one I will remember for the rest of my ride back to Montana.

Guido was full of praise for the people he had met and the country he had seen on his sojourn through the US and was looking forward to meeting many more interesting folks.

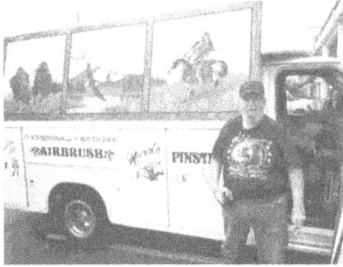

As we visited a man who identified himself as Fuzzy, stepped out of his room and began checking over his truck. He was an artist and was headed to Bike Week to set up his portable paint booth.

He would probably send some bikers home with decorations they didn't expect to have when they rode in.

He also sold paintings he had prepared before leaving his Texas home.

What a talent he showed as we looked over the van which displayed many of his paintings.

The remainder of the trip into Houston was uneventful and a good smooth ride.

SIRI helped me find my way through the suburbs to Richmond where my brother-in-law Stan Smith was ready once again, to offer me a dry and less windy place to stay than the ones I had been used to these past weeks on the road.

17 - Soggy Toll Booth Dollars

We had a great time at dinner the next night with my daughter Joni, her husband Gary and daughter Jerusha, as well as Stan's daughter Shelli, her husband John and son Johnny.

That was a fun evening with many stories to share.

I decided to begin the final leg of my trip from Houston to Lake Mary, Florida a day early.

Always fearful of the Houston week day morning rush hour traffic I took my leave on a Sunday morning.

The Sam Houston Toll Way was one rainy, wet, foggy place to be at 8AM on a Sunday morning.

I had carefully stowed a twenty dollar bill in the side pocket of my rain gear, preparing for the tolls to come. Stopping at the first "pay with change" toll booth I pulled a wet, soggy bill from the rain coat pocket.

"I was trying to keep it dry for you," I called in to the lady who looked somewhat amused at the sight of a dripping wet biker.

She deducted the toll and asked if I would like to have the change wrapped in a paper towel. Nice lady.

 Great idea and she did indeed wrap the change in a couple of paper towels to try and keep it dry for the next toll booth. It did seem to help as I handed the next toll collector a crumpled up wad of paper towels with some not nearly as soggy bills sticking out.

Each toll collector found wetter and wetter paper money, but eventually I had paid the last one and was back on I-10 Eastbound and headed for what I hoped would be warmer, dryer climes.

 The rain and fog stayed with me until I reached the Louisiana border where the first rays of sunshine peeked through a leaden gray sky.

 I was pretty wet, but sunshine helped and Slidell, LA came in to view in early afternoon.

This turned into a beautiful ride through Louisiana.

I pulled into a KOA to make camp.

NO RAIN!

 What a great feeling to have the heater on and things drying out.

Leaving Slidell at 8AM the next morning I prepared for a long day in the saddle.

368 miles to Tallahassee, Florida which would then leave me an easy 240 mile ride to Lake Mary the next day.

I was making good time and pulled in to a Florida Welcome Center to take a break.

 As I dismounted and began removing my helmet I was hailed by a couple who had passed me several miles back. The Harley they were hauling on the trailer would be their ride when they checked in to their Daytona, Florida Bike Week motel.

They were from Austin, Texas and were ready for a big week at Daytona.

Julie, who had seen the 80 Year Old Rider sign on the back of my bike said, "I can't believe you are 80 years old."

Bill said, "Hell man, my bikes on a trailer, I'm only 60 years old and I still can't keep up with you."

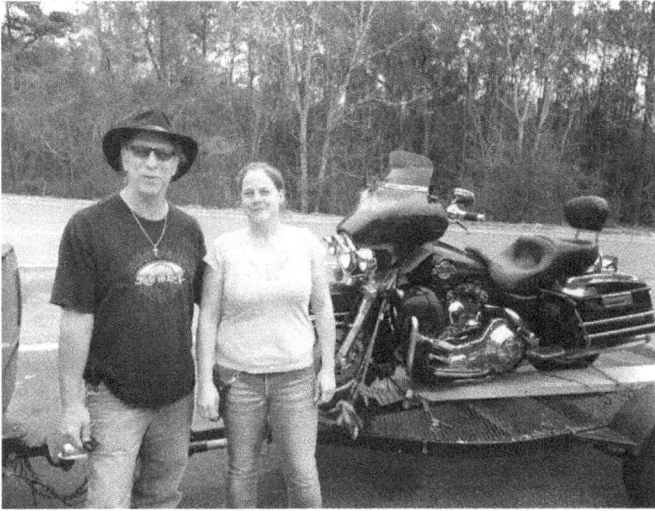

Seems they had passed me a couple of times and each time they got ahead of me they would stop for a break and I would pull ahead of them.

I hope I got their names right, I was so busy visiting I forgot to write them down.

We had a good visit and a couple of laughs and then it was time for me to get back on the road.

The ride south on I-95 was busy but uneventful.

Many bikers were on their way south, heading for a big week in Daytona. Most of them trailering their ride or hauling them in the back of a truck.

Not too many of them riding.

My strange looking rig with sidecar and tent trailer was the object of some bemused looks by visiting bikers.

The biker community is a tight knit group and every time I have had a problem there has been someone there to help, and the two gallon gas can I carry on the back of the sidecar has filled gas tanks for others more often then it has filled mine.

SIRI brought me through the Orlando suburbs and to the driveway of my daughter Diana's home.

Son-in-law Ilidio was there in the driveway to greet me.

It was great to be off the road and relaxing by the pool.

From C 2 C 2 C is the way the Iron Butt Association terms a ride from the Atlantic to the Pacific and back to the Atlantic.

This was the ride I had just completed.

Just not in the time limit necessary to make it an official IBA ride. I rode it as a Flower Sniffer, taking time to enjoy each mile of the way.

What a Grand Adventure.

Now, a few days rest and I would be heading for Denver and then North to Montana.

Life is good and I made it back to Florida in time for a special event being shared with Iron Butt Riders from all over the country.

Ray King's Bike Week RTE (Ride To Eat) for Iron Butt Members at Flagler's Beach, Florida was a great time with many Long Distance Riders to visit with.

THANKS RAY and all others involved in putting together the Bike Week gathering at Martin's Restaurant in Flagler Beach Florida on March 13th.

The crowd gathered early for some tire kicking and war stories about the long rides, the rallies and the good times.

A wide variety of machines rode into the parking lot, many were tricked out with the latest electronics, fuel supplies and Farkels (motorcycle accessories).
The pictures give a quick look at some of the hundred or so riders who attended.

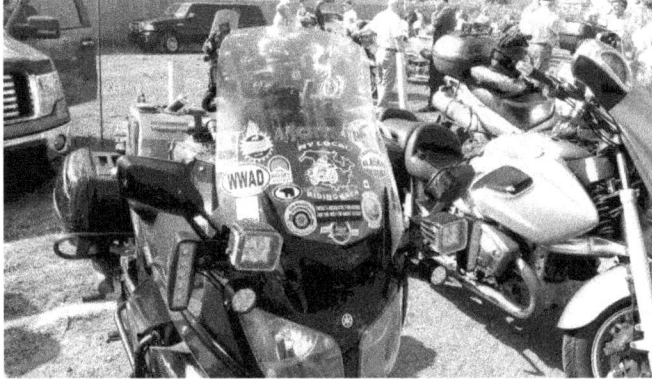

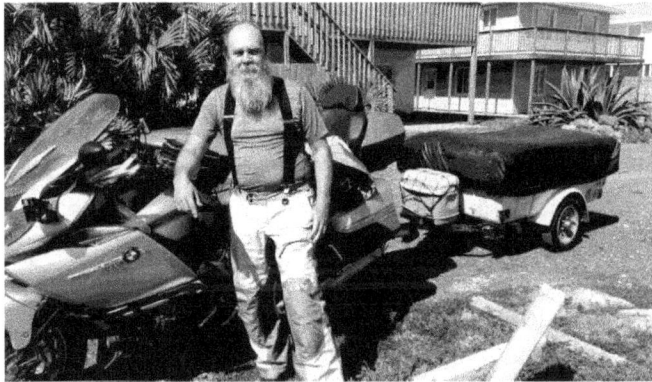

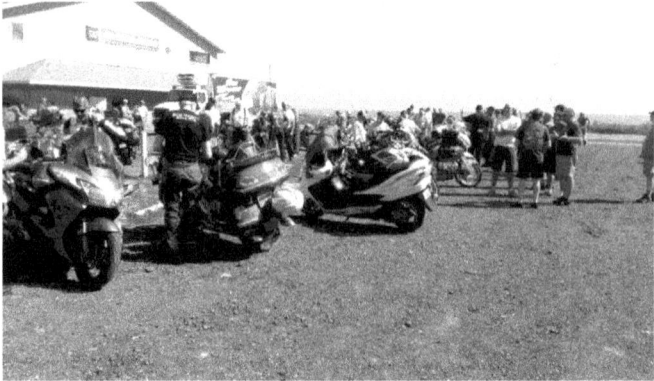

The view from the second floor dining room looked down on the beach and Highway A1A where hundreds of bikers were showing off their machines.

Every kind of bike and riding outfit was on display.
This was a great meet up for Iron Butt Riders.
After lunch and more parking lot visits and many, many tales of long distance rides I was ready to saddle up and get back on the highway.

It was a beautiful day and I turned North to take a longer ride on Florida's famous A1A highway along the coast up to St, Augustine.
Turned south on the interstate and headed back to Lake Mary.
A great way to end a good ride and a great time visiting with Iron Butt Association members from around the USA.
Great people, great country, great day.

18 - Lake Mary To Denver

After enjoying a few more days with Ilidio, before he left for London, I started packing for the trip home.
Where did all this stuff come from?
There seems to be much more than when I started this Grand Adventure Sept. 27, 2014.
I got it all packed, some in the sidecar, the rest in the trailer.
Diana prepared a gourmet seafood snack and spaghetti and meatballs dinner for our last night. It was great. We sat on the lanai, listened to the birds, looked at the Orchid tree and enjoyed the peace and quiet.
Saturday morning, March 21, the first day of spring and the first leg of my four thousand mile ride home to Helena, Montana.
Looks like there could be some rain over toward Alabama so I decided to try and get some miles in and possibly miss the moisture.
Not an Iron Butt ride, but close to it.
Ended the day with 426 miles, plus the extra 40 miles I logged trying to help a stranded biker.
I saw him laying by his bike and looking at something.
I pulled over and said, "looks like you have a problem. Out of gas?"
Young Guy, "No, I have gas, but it starts and runs a short distance and then quits."
I told him I could help if he needed gas, but beyond that I couldn't help.
Ten miles down the road it suddenly dawned on me that I did have an idea that could help and turned around at the next exit and rode the 15 miles back to the last previous exit and found him again.
"Bad Gas," I said, "I had this once when my bike would start and stop like yours."
Both Bill Ryder in Helena and my son-in-law Ilidio had told me to add some fuel stabilizer to the gas tank to prevent this from happening.

Yesterday as I was picking up some last minute camping things I had stopped at Advance Auto supply and picked up a can of Sea Foam additive, which the clerk assured me was the best they had.

I hope it worked for him, I didn't stick around to find out, after all, I was still trying to beat the coming rain.
This extra forty miles running back and forth to try and help had slowed me down.
Of course, if I had thought about it the first time I stopped I could have saved those extra miles, and how many times have I been helped by someone along the road.
Well, we'll see what new adventures tomorrow brings.
This first day could only be described as a great ride.

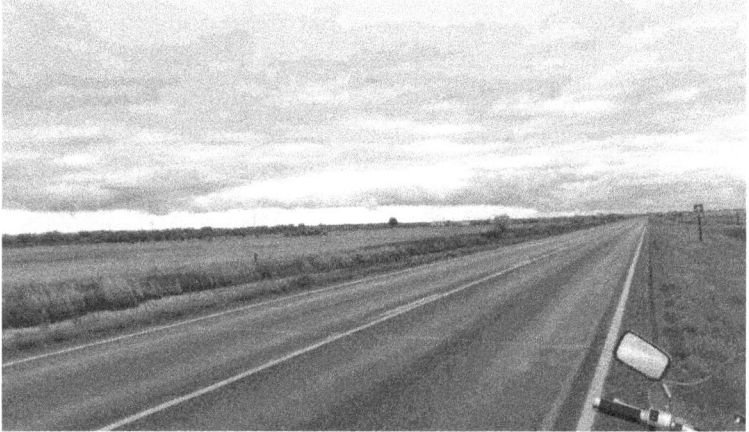

The Long Road

Many, many people passing me along the way waved, smiled and gave the "thumbs up" sign.
They smile at my little sign, and I get to smile back.
We don't seem so much like strangers after that.
This is such a great country.

Yesterdays rain was still hanging in there this morning so my morning 9 AM start was in a light rain.
Light for the first 20 miles.
It then turned into a downpour heavy enough that the "Rest Area 1 mile" sign looked very welcome.

Soaked through despite having all of my rain gear on and with even my "waterproof" boots soaked I walked quickly toward the roofed over, open area of the building.

Seeing another wet biker I said, "Well this wasn't what we wanted to start the day."

Introducing myself I asked about the two very wet Harleys in the parking area.

He said his name was Keith Johnson and he was from Capetown, South Africa.

He and his wife, Corrina, had flown to Miami, rented the bikes and set off on a cross country ride to California and would turn the bikes in at the Los Angeles rental office.

Meanwhile they were drying off and getting ready for their ride to New Orleans.

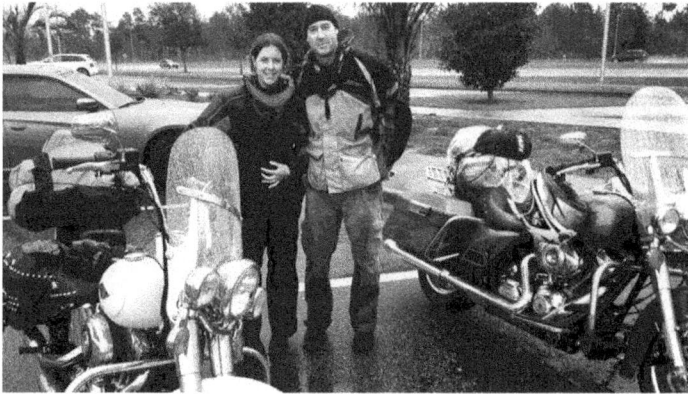

Keith & Corrina Johnson

He took me back to the vending machine area where Corrina had maps spread out so they could check out their travels.

I asked if they had done an Iron Butt ride, which they had not, so I told them to check out IronButt.com and see the many South African IBA members.

They asked about interesting rides and I told them about the Natchez Trace. A great ride after touring New Orleans.

Keith said he was a cabinet maker and they didn't get to ride as often as they would like and were really enjoying their five week vacation in the states.

The rain was letting up a bit and we three headed for our bikes. It was fun visiting with this interesting couple from South Africa. Really nice people and good to see they were enjoying their ride across America.

As I crossed the Alabama state line the sun came out and I was heading into another great ride.
This was a beautiful ride through an area, still wet from the rain.

Seeking a good WiFi spot where I could upload my position on the Facebook page, Where In The World Is Grandpa, and thrill the kids with stories about the great people I was meeting, I pulled into a Wendy's Restaurant.

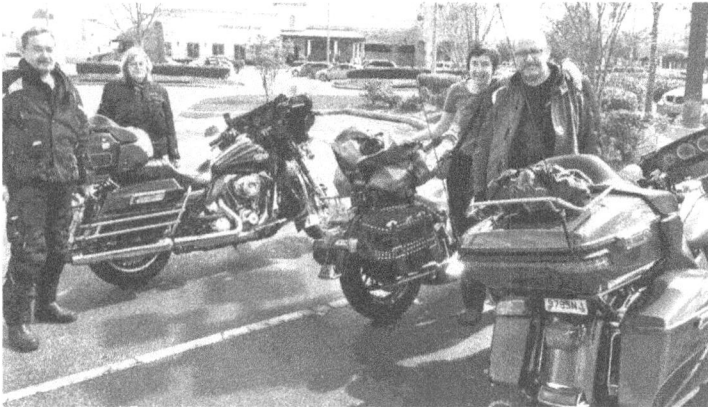

While updating the web page and enjoying a chicken sandwich I saw a group of four bikers arrive and of course went over to their table to introduce myself and see where they were from and where they were heading.
One couple was from Germany and the other from Switzerland.

Like Keith and Corrina, this group had rented bikes in Miami and would return them to a rental office in LA after enjoying a ride across the America. What a great service for these motorcycle rental businesses.
Unfortunately, I tried to use the audio note function on the Iphone6 to get their names.

It didn't work and I don't have their names.
Darned IPhone, or is it just me?
Nice folks and fun to visit with.
Their two week visit will take them coast to coast.
A good ride.

I have had a lot of fun with the "80 year old Iron Butt
Challenge Rider sign on the back of my bike.
Hundreds of people pass me and give me a "Thumbs Up"
as they go by.
Always with a big smile and a wave.
I have fun waving back and with a toot of the horn and big
smile let them know I saw their salute.

Today's experience was a little different, as I rode through
Mississippi.
It happened like this:
A pick up truck with Alabama plates pulled up beside me,
then slowed down and dropped back to get a picture of the
sign. They then completed their pass with big grins and a
wave out the window.
Behind them a large black SUV did the same thing,
although with a new twist I haven't seen before.
The lady passenger didn't have an Iron Butt, she had a very
large Fat Butt.
Which she proved to me as she pulled down her pants and
waved it up and down in the car window as they sped by.
Although a little shocked by this "full window" display, I
did manage a couple of toots on the horn and a friendly
wave.

She poked her hand out and returned the wave, while the
driver almost left the road, apparently in near hysterics at
her actions.

I couldn't hear his laughter, but I could see him slapping
the steering wheel and poking his partner.
They both seemed to have really enjoyed the moment.
No picture to go with this story.
Probably just as well.

I guess when people see other people having a little fun, they just naturally want to join in, even when they don't join in a more traditional manner.

Isn't there a song about this type of thing?

"Mooned Over Mississippi" is the one that comes to mind.

Or is it Moon Over Miami that I'm remembering?

What a great ride today, and tomorrow, the long awaited ride on the Natchez Trace.

Camping was good and the camp site was quiet.

This was a warm night and I had a good nights sleep.

The Grand Adventure continues as I head for home.

Day three of the ride from Florida found me traveling north through Louisiana to reach the starting point of the famous Natchez Trace.

Ever since I read about it in Dale Coyners book on the best rides in North America I had looked forward to doing at least a portion of the Trace.

Time and weather prevented me from riding the entire 499 mile trail, but I did get to go from Natchez to Jackson, Mississippi.

The Natchez Trace is a National Park and I was surprised when the Park Ranger at the headquarters office said she had spent several years in Helena, Montana at the Lewis and Clark National Forest.

Small world indeed.

The Trace was beautiful.

It was springtime as I moved through southern Mississippi with everything turning green and fields of standing water because of the January and February rains.

I stopped at The Waffle House in Jackson, Mississippi for a late breakfast and was surprised when a guy sitting at the counter said he was from Miles City, Montana.

We had to talk for a moment about the annual Bucking Horse Sale for which Miles City is famous.

After leaving the Natchez Trace National Park scenic drive at Jackson, Mississippi I headed North on I-55.

This was a great ride with good highway, light traffic and sunshine filled skies. I was riding in a light west wind. Just enough breeze to keep it cool and comfortable. With just one brief stop at a McDonald's to update the WITWIG Facebook group, I pulled into the Frog Hollow Campgrounds in Grenada, Mississippi at 5:30 pm.

Although I had ridden in beautiful sunshine the last few hours, the camp grounds were soggy having received over five inches of rain the day before. As I made my way toward my designated Camping site I got stuck in the mud surrounding it and had to be pushed into the parking spot.

I guess I shouldn't have revved up the Yamaha engine while the guys were behind me pushing. The rear wheel sort of sprayed them with mud from head to toe. Boy were they muddy. But we got it in and they forgave me for the mess. The set up was quick, not many RVers wanting to look the rig over. The sun was shining next morning as I pulled out of the Frog Hollow camp grounds and headed north on I-55. But I was riding with a cold Northeast wind all the way up to Memphis, Tennessee. I suppose I should have done the touristy thing and looked for Graceland, but instead I cruised right on through and headed for Cape Girardeau, Missouri. My gas stop in Osceola, Arkansas just before noon was quick and the obligatory stop at McDonald's to use their WiFi to update WITWIG and then I was back on the road heading for Cape Girardeau.

That blasted Northeast wind seemed to be getting stronger and colder as I rode north on I-55 and I pulled off at Sikeston, Missouri, thirty five miles short of Cape G. The rain was just starting to come down and I pulled into the parking lot of the first motel I came to. It was a Comfort Inn. Good choice and it was good to get settled in to a nice warm room. The next morning started out sunny but cool. A great day for a ride.

The 150 miles to St. Louis went by quickly and by mid-morning I was moving with the heavy flow of traffic around the city on I-270. As the by-pass route turned north on the west side of the city I was feeling comfortable despite the heavy traffic.

At the beginning of this book I described an accident and this was the spot where it happened.

Everything was going along smoothly and I was about to move off I-270 and onto I-70 west when without warning the young man driving in lane one drifted to the right and hit three barrels of sand being used as a construction site barricade. As the Four lane highway was about to become a three lane road and with heavy traffic moving at 70 mph the excitement was about to begin.

The young guy slammed on his brakes and began skidding sideways across all four lanes.

I was in lane three and hit the brakes hard.

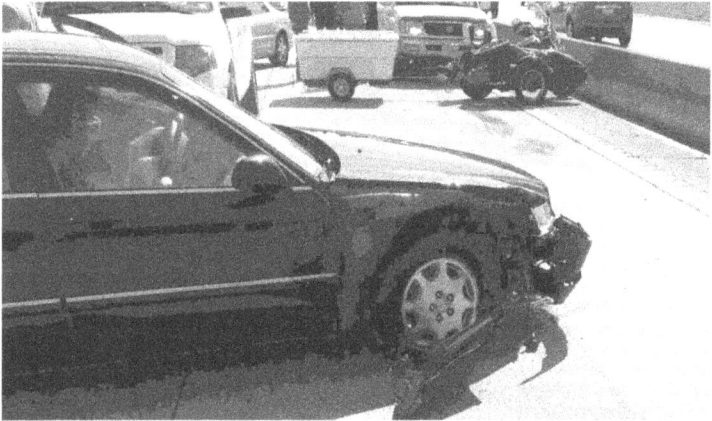

As his car swerved across the road it and we were about to make contact, the car in lane two swerved to the left and T-Boned the kid on the drivers side door.

That pushed him away from me and I skidded to a stop, still sideways, almost touching the concrete barrier.

I thought he was going to get me but driver two collided with him first and saved me from being part of the crash.

The young guy driving the pick up truck behind me managed to stop quickly enough to avoid hitting me.

When we were all stopped he came running over shouting "Are you all right? Are you all right?"
I told him I was fine.
He said "mister I don't care how old you are that was one helluva a piece of riding you just did. When you started jack knifing I thought you were a goner. Great ride Mister, Great ride. "
The good part about the entire episode was of course the fact that no one was hurt. The young man who started the whole thing was pretty shook up, but otherwise not injured. I checked the bike over to see if the quick, skidding stop had caused any damage to the struts which hold the sidecar in place. Everything was fine.

As we waited for the police, whose sirens could be heard in the distance, I told the young pick up truck driver that I could back away from the concrete barrier and clear the lane so we could get traffic moving in at least that one lane.

Semi trucks and cars were already backed up as far back as we could see.

As I pulled away several of the other drivers shouted Good Bye and Be Safe all the while giving the familiar thumbs up sign.

There was no traffic ahead of me or behind me.
I was alone on the road and alone with my thoughts.

"Faith, you just have to have faith." Lois would have said. She showed her faith in many ways.
One day Linda was reading from the Stories of Great Hymns book, that Janis had sent her Mom.
Lois, who hadn't spoken in several weeks looked her in the eye and said, "You know that's true don't you?"
Linda said later, "Janis really hit the mark when she sent this book with stories about Mom's favorite hymns.
She listens so intently to each story."

As we did evening prayers I was never quite sure whether she understood what we were doing, until one night, I decided to repeat the prayer we said with the kids all those years ago, when they were very young.
"God Bless Mom and Dad, God Bless Allen and Linda, God Bless Diana and Janis, God Bless Joni and Roger and so on.
By the time I reached Allen and Linda, Lois reached over and laid her hand on mine, as if to say, "I remember and I understand."
No words were spoken, but the message was there.
It was one of many very touching moments.
What does she understand? What does she remember?
What memories are playing back in her mind?
Questions many others have asked.
Touching moments many other care givers have felt while making their own journey through this strange illness.

   Well, the accident in St. Louis is now one more little adventure to tell the kids about.
I was pretty calm throughout the actual event, but as I rode on, nerves were jangling and the many thoughts going through my mind were probably moving faster then me and my bike were moving down the interstate.
I wasn't tired this afternoon and kept riding and thinking. In fact, like that battery bunny we see on TV, I just kept going and going.
Making it a long days ride until I ended up at the High Plains Camp Ground in Oakley, Kansas, some 600 miles from my early morning starting point at Sikeston, Missouri. Maybe that little near miss in St. Louis affected me more than I thought.

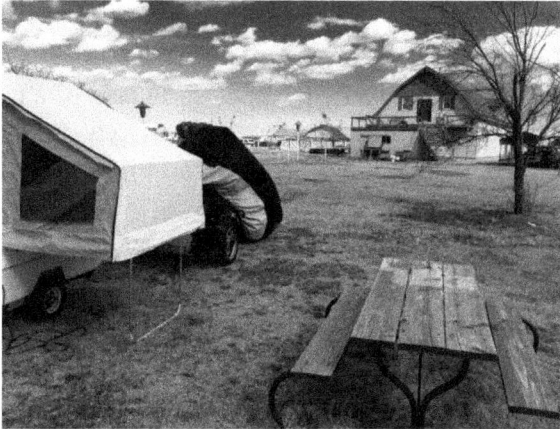

High Plains Camp Ground - Oakley, Kansas

Camping at the High Plains Campgrounds in Oakley,
Kansas was another good experience.
I was way out on the Kansas prairie at a crossroads camp.
It had been a sunny, windy and cool ride across that part of
the state. Lots of wind farms, oil wells, and cattle.
Clouds were drifting across an endless sky and birds were
everywhere. Their songs filled the air.
The wind died down and after a dinner break at the
Captains Lounge and a genuine Oakley Burger I called it a
day.
   I have to admit, sleep was a long time coming.
The excitement of the day took awhile to settle down.
"All is well that ends well," my Mother used to say, and I
guess that would certainly apply to this days adventure.
Should make Denver tomorrow, if the weather holds.
We'll see what great adventures await.
It will be good to see Jarred, Malachi and Ashley again.
Grandkids are the greatest.

19 - Denver - The Snooze Eatery & Home

Pulled into a Denver Super 8, instead of a campgrounds so I could be closer to downtown Denver and the restaurant that Diana had told her son Jared to take me to when I visited his city.

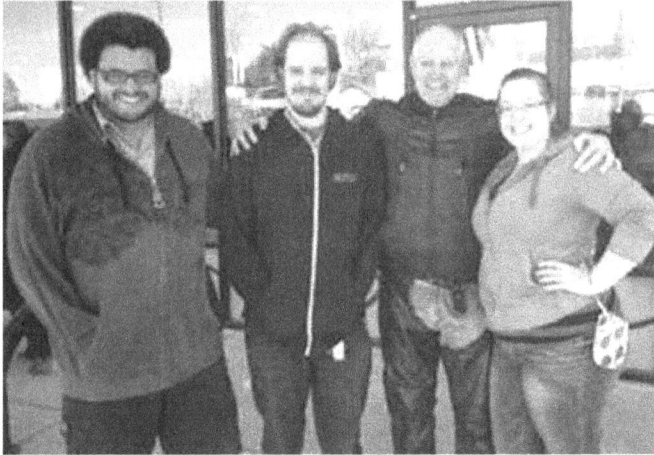

I arrived an hour early for breakfast the next morning, since I wasn't sure if SIRI would get me to this highly recommended breakfast spot called The Snooze Eatery. The parking lot was jammed, even at 8AM and I had to circle the block waiting for a space to open up. Service must be good because the parking spaces emptied and filled on a regular basis. One trip around the lot and I had a spot. As I was getting off the bike a car stopped behind me as if waiting for me to leave, I smiled and said, "Sorry folks I just got here."
The woman responded, "It's okay, we just stopped so the kids could see your motorcycle."
It does seem to attract attention.
Inside I was told there would be a 35 to 55 minute wait. WOW! This place is really good.
I waited on the street outside with other would-be-breakfast-eaters and by 8:30AM I saw Joni's son Malachi and wife Ashley coming, both with big welcoming smiles.

Jared arrived a short time later and we had a good visit and even got a guy from Virginia to take a couple of pictures. The breakfast was unique at this well known upscale breakfast spot.

Eggs cooked in every way known to man, including great Mexican and Oriental styles.

Great food and a wonderful visit with three young people who are living their dream in what they believe to be the best city in the country.

Leaving the restaurant we found a group of half a dozen people gathered around my rig in the parking lot.

One of them turned out to be from Whitefish, Montana. They saw the rig and wanted to look closer at it, asking questions about the sidecar and Mini Mate trailer, and of course had a good laugh when they saw the 80 year old biker sign.

Putting a smile on the face of a stranger, what could be more fun than that?

And the sign has done that hundreds of times during the course of my trek across the country.

SIRI took me directly out of town on I-25 North and I was soon on my way, while still remembering and enjoying the stories and laughter of my visit with the Denver grand kids.

Casper Wyoming was the goal and I made it in good time. The only campground in town that I could find didn't look all that great so I opted for the Comfort Inn.

Good choice, this was a well cared for motel and I got a good nights sleep.

What a great day, beginning with the Denver Grands and continuing with a great ride north on I-25. Colorado has a lot of friendly people and many of them waved, honked their horns and gave a thumbs up as I rode through their state. Thanks Colorado.

Leaving Casper, I thought I would stop for the night in Billings, Montana so I lingered over breakfast longer then I should have and didn't get on the road until 9AM.

Strong head winds and those Wyoming hills slowed my rig and I was getting a good upper arm workout, but the ride went well with short gas stops and long rides in between. Running low on fuel I was looking for a gas station and saw a sign that said KayCee, Wyoming, fuel and food, and then a sign that said "Chris Ledoux Memorial Park."

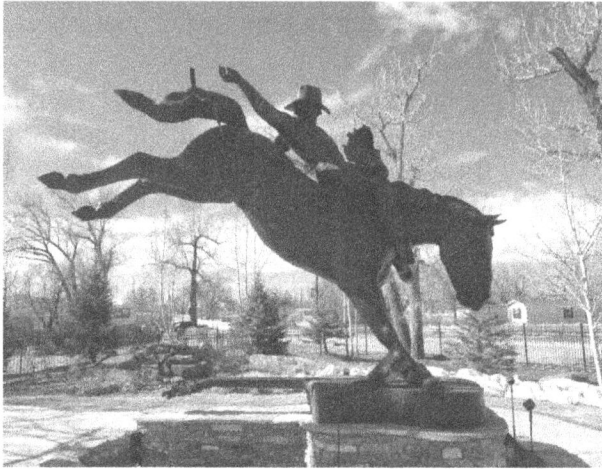

Way out here, in the middle of Wyoming a park honoring Chris Ledoux? Wow! This I had to see.

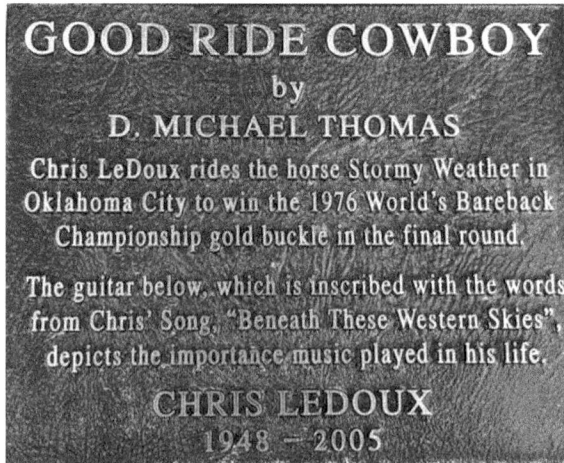

GOOD RIDE COWBOY
by
D. MICHAEL THOMAS

Chris LeDoux rides the horse Stormy Weather in Oklahoma City to win the 1976 World's Bareback Championship gold buckle in the final round.

The guitar below, which is inscribed with the words from Chris' Song, "Beneath These Western Skies", depicts the importance music played in his life.

CHRIS LEDOUX
1948 – 2005

Filled the gas tank and drove down the street a couple of blocks and there it was, a life size bronze statue of Chris Ledoux riding a horse called Stormy Weather to the 1976World Bareback Bronc Riding Championship. Chris was known to sing his cowboy songs at every rodeo he competed in, and had even made a couple of cassette recordings that he sold along the way.

When Garth Brooks released a record in which he sang about "listening to a worn out tape of Chris Ledoux," Chris was off on a new career as a country music star.

Some day when you're on a long ride through Wyoming and you see a sign that says, "Kaycee, Wyoming" you might want to pull off the interstate and visit a great park and maybe meet some nice folks.

Making good time I arrived in Billings at 2PM and decided to ride straight through to Helena without the planned lay over.

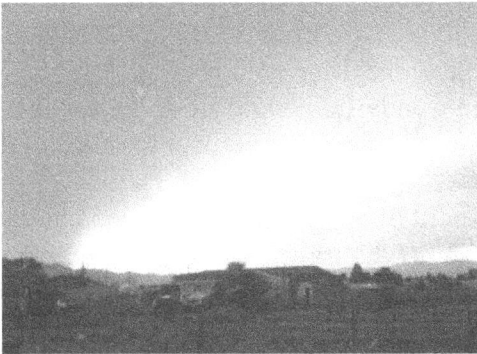

It would take only four more hours in the saddle. The wind had died down a little and it was a good ride. Smoke from the weekend fires between Laurel and Park City was still visible but the Interstate was open and I made good time. Even the construction project near Toston didn't slow me down much. 7:30 PM and I sent a text to Roger to let him know I was coming into Helena and heading for Perkins for a good dinner. He came and we ate and we talked about the ride. It felt good to be back in familiar surroundings.

I rode into the driveway and I was home.
It felt very good.

Linda met me at the house with all the mail she had been saving for me and it was good to be home.

It was March 30 and the odometer told me I had traveled 16,264 miles on the Yamaha since leaving Helena at 4AM on the morning of September 27th.

Six months and 16,000 miles.

The 12 months total mileage since the day Lois had passed away was 26,369 miles.

This has been an epic adventure visiting interesting places and meeting interesting people, and making many new friends.

It had started with the thousand mile Iron Butt ride to Minneapolis and there I turned in to what the Long Distance Riders call a "Flower Sniffer."

I stopped to smell the flowers many times along the way.

This ride is not over yet.

We didn't choose to live this life without Lois, but we can choose to live it fully and live it well.

I do believe that is just what Lois would have wanted.

There are miles to go, wondrous things to see, and most important, people to meet.

I have met some wonderful people along the way and have found an America that has great respect for it's elderly citizens.

And most important of all, the children, grand children and great grand children who traveled with Lois and I on the journey through Alzheimer's Disease, and with me on a 26,000 mile motorcycle ride across the country have discovered, as I have, there is indeed

Life After Alzheimer's!

Lois knew that.
She knew there would be life for her family after her journey through Alzheimer's Disease was complete.
As she moved slowly from one stage of the illness to another, she talked about the problems she was having doing things she wanted to get done.
She struggled hard and became frustrated as these every day tasks became ever more difficult.
At some point during this period she wrote a song, which I found on her computer, months after she was gone.
I think she meant for me to find it like that.
We had performed together for sixty years, and now in the words of a song, she left me one last message.

Keep on singing and do it with pride and joy.

She called it: "When You Sing Your Song"

When You Sing Your Song
Lois Lonnquist

When you sing your song, sing it happy
Add some notes of harmony,
Stand up proud - before the crowd,
in the background you'll hear me.
chorus
You'll still hear me, singing harmony,
Yes, you'll still hear me, singing harmony

Remember the years, we sang our songs,
So sweet in memory
We stood up proud - before the crowd,
And presented our shows, you and me.
chorus
You'll still hear me, singing harmony,
Yes, you'll still hear me, singing harmony

When the time comes you'll solo again
In the days that soon will be,
Still stand up proud - before the crowd,
And from somewhere, you'll hear me.
chorus
You'll still hear me, singing harmony,
Yes, you'll still hear me, singing harmony

She was right again.
I pick up a guitar, strum a few chords, start to sing,
and there she is.
I do hear her singing that same old harmony.

There is
Life After Alzheimer's Disease.

Sing your song and sing it happy.

Some of the things
that worked for us as Caregivers

  The journey through Alzheimer's Disease is unique to each individual.

  Caregivers are often faced with questions for which there are no answers in books or on the internet and will often face situations they haven't read about or heard about from other care givers.

  The ideas, comments and suggestions on the following pages may provide some insight into caregiving for dementia patients, as seen from one family who successfully completed the journey.

  One of the things I have not seen discussed or written about is Role Reversal. Advance preparation for the role of caregiver and house keeper would have been a great benefit.

  Like many other husbands, I thought I had helped out a lot around the house. But as I took over more and more household duties and I began to realize how much Lois had always done I could see many area where I could have been of more help. Helping around the house more would have made the role reversal much easier!
Spouses should help each other prepare for the Role Reversal that will take place when one of them is gone.

  Don't be hesitant in asking for help. Family and friends are often at a loss as to what they can do. TELL THEM! Remember, people want to help and you are doing them a favor by letting them know of specific ways to be of service. Even small breaks are important for the health of the primary caregiver.

Don't be afraid to ask your Health Care Professional about hospice. Hospice programs provide assistance and information invaluable for the caregiver.

Frontier Hospice of Helena, Montana has a wonderful, caring staff who provided many services, suggestions and ideas which made Lois' journey through this insidious disease more bearable. For these wonderful people we have only our deepest gratitude.

Hospice may provide a bath person to help with bathing. Having the Hospice Bath Lady lifted a big burden from Linda as she had been coming from her night nursing job at the VA Hospital to help Lois with her bath three mornings a week. The bath ladies were wonderful. Once a routine was established Lois looked forward to seeing them.

We were able to add to that by hiring a podiatry nurse to give Lois a pedicure on a regular basis. She did wonders while trimming toe nails and doing a foot massage. Lois had always had some problems with her feet and this special care was a great comfort to her and to us. For people with diabetes or arthritis podiatry is especially important.

Consider hiring someone to come in and assist with housework. Even having the bathrooms, kitchen and vacuuming done frees a lot of hours per month to spend caregiving and removes a level of stress.

At every stage of dementia physical contact is important: Hold hands, brush hair, use lotion on hands and feet for dry skin. While they are still mobile take them on walks and car rides. A word of caution, people with dementia can be impulsive and car doors should have electric locks. While riding with one of her daughters Lois accidently opened a door that had manual locks.

Dementia brings paranoia and leads to hiding of treasurers

in strange places. Be aware of things disappearing and watch for places where they can be hidden.

   Invite friends and relatives to visit. Encourage them to do the things they have always enjoyed, even if it needs to be modified or done on a smaller scale.
   Reading is important for many people. Lois very much enjoyed the time spent with family reading to her. If you are unable to read to them personally contact your state's Talking Book Library For The Blind or Disabled.
They will provide talking books at no charge.
   Include your loved one in every way, even if they no longer seem to understand and can't respond in the way you expect. Talk to them, not about them when standing by their chair or bed with other people.
   In the late stages we placed Lois's hospital bed in the Living Room and pointed it out from the corner toward the center of the room. The kids decorated her surroundings for each holiday and special occasion.
  When we had guests visiting, she was included in the conversation, whether she could take part or not. Someone was always at her side when there was company giving her added security and comfort.
   Socializing with family and friends is important in all stages of dementia.
   Joni came from Houston, TX and stayed for weeks at a time providing breaks for the caregiver and singing and reading to her Mom. When she was unable to come personally she provided songs over the internet and Facebook. Janis came several times from San Jose, CA, and spent time talking, singing and reading to her Mom while she was visiting.
   Janice came two days a week during those last two years and provided many hours out of the house for me. She often put a Netflix movie on or brought a DVD so they could watch a movie together. She also enjoyed feeding

pistachio pudding to Lois and holding her hand after she was no longer capable of speech.

Hanna and Lorna, along with their children, also sang in person and over the internet. Lois enjoyed time watching her great grandchildren playing.

These hours spent together are a time of special closeness and preparing for the future for parent, children, grandchildren and friends. This type of involvement by family members was key to keeping Lois entertained and involved.

As the primary care giver I was not forgotten as I received frequent phone calls from Allen, Ilidio and others from out-of-state. Even when Lois was no longer able to participate, these calls were another important way of giving me a break from the daily routines.

Roger was always available for coffee at the Donut Hole or Perkins. During the Alzheimer's journey it is important to remember the health of the primary caregiver is essential to both caregiver and care receiver.

People with dementia are easily overwhelmed by noise, people and new situations. They may be unable to shop, go to movie or go out to eat in the later stages.

Don't offer too many choices at once. You may need to pick out clothing for them. Put small amounts of food on their plate as even too much food can be a sensory overload. Just play it by ear. If they seem anxious then it may be time to make another adjustment.

Although your loved one may not be able to express their desires about personal appearance it is still important to them.

We were fortunate to find a wonderful lady who came to the house and gave Lois a permanent once every four months. Lois loved it and it made caring for her hair easier.

Clothing needs change through the various stages of Alzheimer's. As the disease goes from early to moderate many people unbutton, unsnap and unzip clothing at inappropriate times. During this stage try using elastic waist band pants and pull- over shirts. Body heat regulation may be an issue and sweat suits work well for many people.
During the early moderate stage of the disease, most clothing had zippers in front which made changing easier.
   As the disease progressed and she was confined to the hospital bed, clothing was cut down the back with ties attached at the neck.
   Janis and Mike sent us a gift certificate from The Vermont Country Store and I ordered a beautiful red, lacey floor length dress. Linda cut it down the back and added ties so that even when she was confined to her bed, slipping her into this beautiful dress was easy to do. When company came she looked very nice, as she would have wanted.

   Security is important and needs will change as the disease progresses. Pre-planning can make this process easier as changes occur.
   Diana and Ilidio came from Florida and installed a large awning over an enclosed deck, making it possible for Lois to go outside and still be in a safe and secure place. She spent a lot of time that summer on the deck watching the deer and the birds.
   Aaron and Hanna built and installed a heavy, lockable gate on the lower level staircase. Although she tried, she was never able to figure out the lock and was kept safe from the stairway.

Roger and Janice found a loud alarm that would sound if she opened any of the exterior doors. It startled her and for a time kept her from trying to go out.

I installed children's safety locks on cupboard doors and plastic locks on closet doors. We were not very successful in keeping her out of closets. She would jerk on the door until the lock broke. There must be a better way.

Often people with dementia develop a shuffling gait, so area rugs and other potential dangers should be removed or adjusted.

Nutrition is important, but can be one of the most challenging issues in moderate and later stages of Alzheimer's.

In moderate stages small amounts of favorite foods often are not as overwhelming and the taste is familiar. One study we read suggested using a red plate because sometimes with dementia there can be visual problems and the red plate helps to distinguish the food easier. We tried it, but never determined if it really worked.

Because of another health problem, Systemic Scleroderma , Lois was unable to easily swallow food. This is often a problem in later stages of dementia as well.

After much research of nutrition sites on line we developed what we called The "Super Shake" which she received four times a day. The thick liquid consistency made it easier to swallow.

It consisted of :

1 bottle of Ensure Nutrition drink
1 serving (quarter cup) of Ricotta Cheese
1 serving (half a cup) of ice cream
1 scoop of Whey Protein powder

We mixed this in a blender, added her crushed up prescription drugs and gave it to her with a straw. She always loved Dairy Queen milk shakes, so this was readily accepted.

Her weight had dropped to 97 pounds. In a few short months on the Super Shake she was over 120 pounds. The shake provided 450 calories, so for several months she received 1800 calories per day. We then began cutting back and continually adjusted the amounts right up until her final days.

Tall plastic glasses with lids and straws that have stoppers on them are a good idea to prevent spills and messes. They are available at any discount store and come in many fun and bright patterns. Janice and Linda both purchased some of these easy to clean glasses.

During the early to moderate stages of the disease taking her medications on time was a problem. We designed a "Pill Page" which had color pictures and names of each pill along with times each medication was due. This way Lois could look at the page taped to the cupboard door where her pills were kept and by looking at the picture of the pill know which one to take.

During the moderate stages we used a pill box with removable strips for each day. This allowed us to remove one day at a time and keep the rest of the pills locked in the cupboard. The pill box not only kept Lois from taking an overdose of meds, but also allowed all the caregivers to see what had been given and what was still due. It also allowed her to continue to participate in medication administration. This worked for many months, but as cognitive abilities faded different methods were needed and we began crushing the pills between two soup spoons and adding them to her Super Shake.

Hospice can assist with setting up medications if caregivers are unsure about doing it themselves.

Be aware of negative side effects of some Alzheimer's medications. Early on Lois did have one bad reaction to a medication and we watched closely all medications and her reaction to them. It is good to check potential side effects with doctors, nurses and pharmacists.

As a family we were always looking for things that would provide brain stimulation and fun.
For these things consider prior employment and activities the person enjoyed.
Lois always loved music so we used the Pandora on line music service which played through our computer and TV. We chose Slack Key Guitar lullabies as background music. It played through the TV and provided hours of soothing music for $36.00 per year. This service is free if you don't mind listening to an occasional commercial.
If you haven't tried Slack Key Guitar, look for it on You Tube, Pandora, Itunes etc. Very soothing music.

Lois enjoyed sewing before dementia. Now she spent hours using children's lacing shapes to "sew." The heavy cardboard shapes had holes around the edges into which she could thread colorful yarn.
Linda made a "Fabric Book" out of different types of fabric. This provided both visual and sensory stimulation. Lois would hold the book in her lap, turn the pages and run her hands across the material on each page. She would hold this book in her lap for hours even in the late stages.

Lift the flap Fisher Price children's board books and wooden jig saw puzzles that had with pieces with knobs were easy to handle. Linda bought a board with many different kinds of locks on it was found in a toy department.
Because of her experience as a reporter, author and researcher she enjoyed large forms and papers she could

fill out with a pen or pencil. This worked through the moderate stages of the disease.

 Having raised six children Lois loved babies and small children. A picture book with photos of family members gave her pleasure in the early and early/moderate stages.
 Years earlier Linda had given Lois two collector dolls dressed in cowboy suits.
She had them stored away in a closet. As the illness progressed we got the dolls out and Linda found baby outfits for them to wear. Lois loved holding and talking to them. One day she said to Linda, "Jack is such a sweet little boy, but he doesn't say much."
They were a part of her life for many months.
 These dolls from the Adora Doll Company are weighted and are the size of a newborn baby.

 In the late stages, when Lois was mostly confined to bed, everything necessary for her care was stored on small shelving units which for many years had held her books, CD's and DVD's. They stood against the walls on either side of her bed, within easy reach of caregivers.

 The TAP - Turning And Positioning System made moving her around while she was being changed or being moved to the recliner much easier. It was purchased from Sage Medical Systems on line. Other companies may have similar systems. This unit made it possible for me to move her around on the bed and from the bed to the recliner by myself without causing skin tears or bed sores, and saving my back by making lifting and turning much easier. It is a Caregiver Lifesaver, or at least it was for Lois and I.

 An air filled mattress pad which circulated air back and forth as she lay on it was invaluable for making sure that she never had a bed sore or any other skin problems. It was available through Hospice, paid for by Medicare and rented from a local medical supply store.

   Disposable underwear, both pull up and with taped sides also save a lot of time and laundry. Baby wipes are great for keeping skin clean and infection free.
   Oral care is important even after the person is no longer able to brush their teeth." Toothettes" and mouthwash that can be swallowed are a good way to keep the mouth clean to prevent infections. Toothettes and wipes are available through Hospice and also online.

   Skin care and monitoring is vital with a bedbound person. Keep skin clean and dry. Make sure clothing and bedding is clean and wrinkle free.
Get advice for any pink areas or open sores.

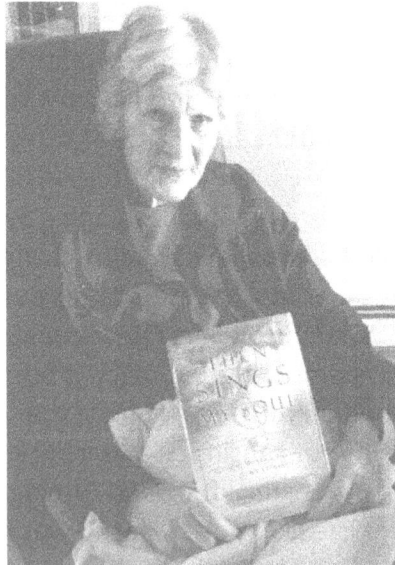

Lois with favorite hymn book

During the final week of her life our children gathered around her bed, and as they had done so many years earlier, they sang to her in four part harmony. The hymns and folk songs provided a soothing , caring, loving period for all of the family.

Great Hymns to carry her home.

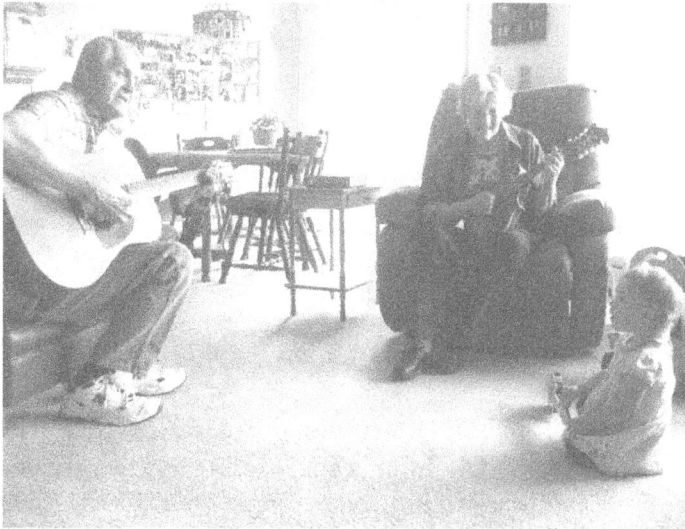

Del, Lois and Great Grand Daughter Liliana
Lois loved music and children

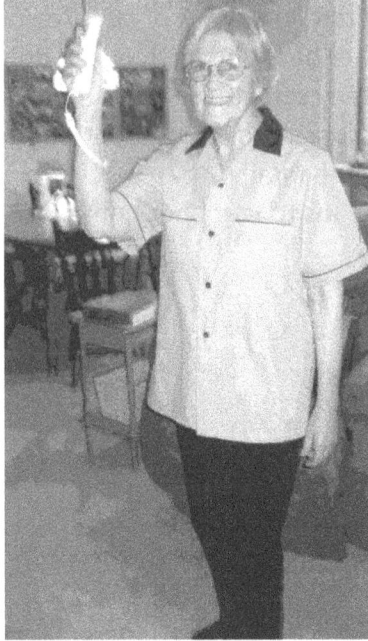

**Wii Bowling was great exercise until
Alzheimer's Disease brought confusion
and inability to operate the controls**

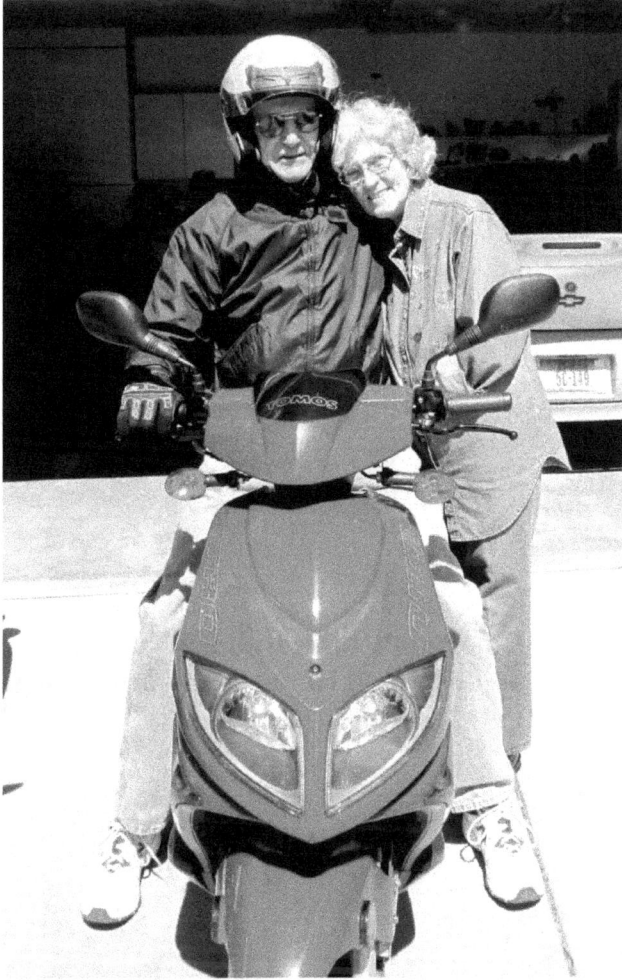

Lois and Del
before the Alzheimer's decline became apparent

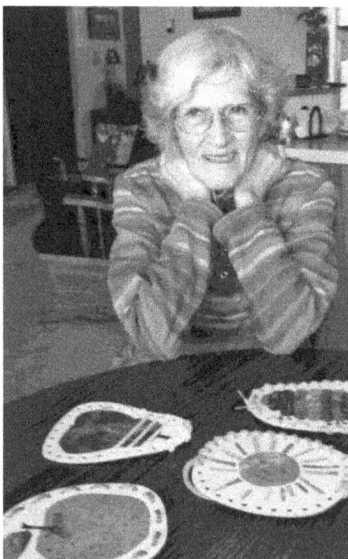

**Colorful Pictures with holes around the edges
so Lois could lace colored yarn through them**

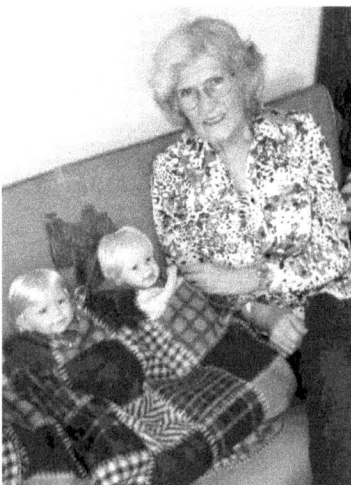

The always present large dolls, Jack & Jill

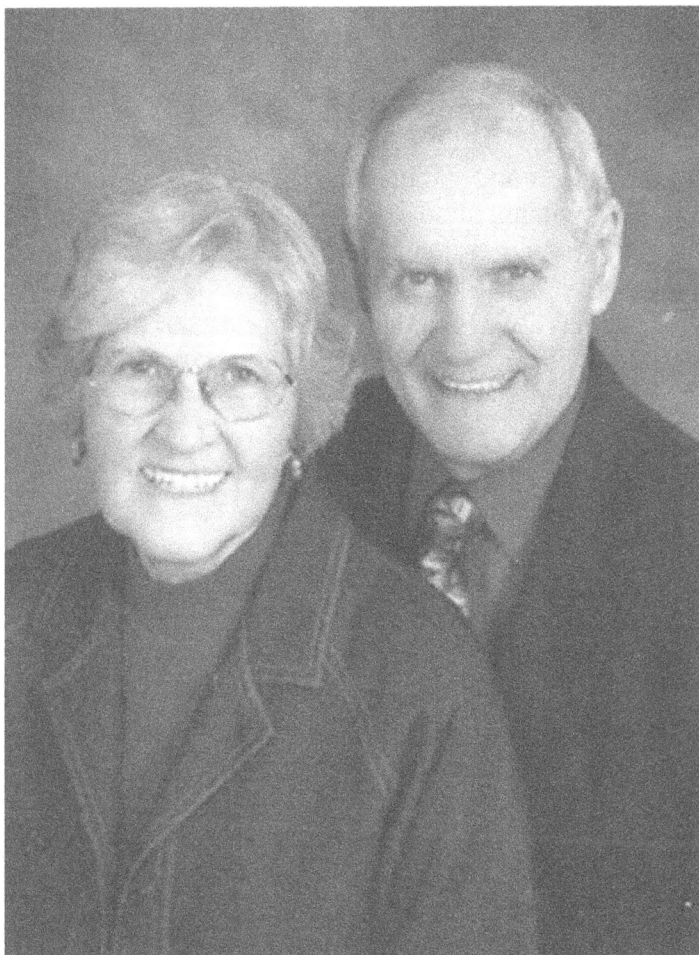

Lois & Del Before Alzheimer's Disease

ABOUT THE AUTHOR

Del Lonnquist worked in broadcasting for over 40 years, working at radio stations as a dee jay, news reporter, manager and station owner.
He took his family to live in several states from Minnesota, Wisconsin, Michigan, Florida and Montana.

He has always ridden motorcycles and had a passion for long distance riding.

When Lois passed away three weeks before their 60th anniversary he took to the road as therapy and to become reconciled to his new life.
In the 12 months after her death he rode 26,000 miles.
His travels took him from Washington state to Washington DC from Montana to Florida and from Florida to California.
He met many people, visited children, grand children and great grandchildren and thought a lot about Lois.
In this book he attempts to express some of those thoughts.